What Are You Feeling, Doctor?

Identifying and avoiding defensive patterns in the consultation

John Salinsky

and

Paul Sackin

Foreword by
Dame Lesley Southgate
*Professor of Primary Care and Medical Education,
Royal Free and University College Medical School, London*

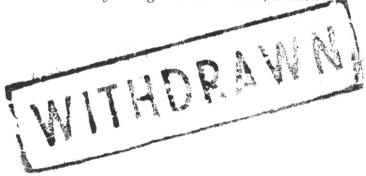

Radcliffe Medical Press

© 2000 John Salinsky and Paul Sackin

Radcliffe Medical Press Ltd
18 Marcham Road, Abingdon, Oxon OX14 1AA

British Library Cataloguing in Publication Data

A catalogue record for this book is available from the British Library.

ISBN 1 85775 407 7

Typeset by Action Publishing Technology, Gloucester
Printed and bound by TJ International Ltd, Padstow, Cornwall

Contents

Foreword

In the early 1970s I joined a Balint group. During the next 5 years, a period of full-time busy general practice for me, I began to make sense of the consultation. But the greatest benefit came from hearing the stories of doctor–patient relationships recounted by other group members. They brought my own relationships with patients into sharp, and sometimes uncomfortable, focus. I can recall those sessions very clearly 25 years later and in particular my private learning about my own defences. Those lessons had to be learned over and over again, as consultations apparently straightforward became unpredictable and dysfunctional.

Communication between patients and doctors is analysed, debated and assessed in modern general practice more than ever before. Assessment of video-taped consultations is mandatory before a doctor can commence independent practice in the UK. In the USA there is a formal requirement to evaluate the humanistic behaviour of internal medicine residents, including the qualities of integrity, respect and compassion. But although the expectations of doctors' behaviour are explicit, things can still go wrong. Sometimes the doctor's feelings get in the way.

In this book the work of a traditional Balint group is extended beyond its previous boundaries. Starting from the patient's story and the recounting of the doctor–patient relationship, the reader is allowed to meet the personal self of the doctor. The feelings and defences of the doctor are explored. General practitioners will recognise the authenticity of the work of the group. Others will gain more understanding of the apparently perverse behaviour of some doctors with some patients. But the analytical part of the book takes us beyond description on to analysis and reflection about what might be done. The implications for future research and reforms in medical education are considerable. This work for the future will also mark the joining together of the Balint group method with approaches such as evidence-based medicine and the assessment of clinical competence. The missing pieces about the failure of some doctors to incorporate best practice into the consultation may be addressed by paying attention to what the doctor is feeling rather than what he/she knows.

Professor Dame Lesley Southgate
May 2000

Preface

Although family doctors are now trained in communication skills and encouraged to study their interactions with their patients on video, there are still too many consultations which leave both doctor and patient feeling troubled. This is likely to occur when the patient arouses disturbing feelings in the doctor which are not recognised or understood. Unable to cope with these feelings, doctors often develop powerful defence mechanisms to protect themselves. Some defences are essential if the doctor is to survive and to continue to function professionally. But excessive and unnecessary defences simply prevent him from listening with empathy. In this situation the doctor knows perfectly well what to do to achieve a successful consultation, but finds himself unable to do it because he can no longer 'tune in' to the patient's feelings.

This book is based on the work of a group of general practitioners who met regularly over a 5-year period to explore the defensive over-reactions and failures of empathy which they noted in their everyday consultations. The process of working was based on the well-known 'Balint' method of case discussion. This was originally developed by Michael Balint, a psychiatrist and psychoanalyst who worked with groups of general practitioners in London in the 1950s and 1960s to study the dynamics of doctor–patient relationships.

Our group consisted of ten experienced general practitioners, two of whom acted as group leaders or facilitators. The group members presented case histories in which they had felt confused, disturbed or upset either during or after the consultation. After each presentation the group examined what was going on in the doctor–patient relationship, looking in particular for evidence that the doctor was using defences of some sort to protect himself from engaging emotionally with the patient. We discovered that emotional withdrawal can happen with lightning speed before the doctor realises what is happening. We recognised that some of these defensive withdrawals were necessary to preserve the doctor's ability to function. But we also found that many defences were excessive and inappropriate, denying doctor and patient the opportunity to share feelings in a therapeutic way.

We evolved a series of questions to help us to understand what was going on. We wanted to know, in particular, whether the patient's presentation 'would have upset other doctors' or whether the defences were mobilised because the patient's feelings resonated with something painful in that particular doctor's personal history. This led us to explore our own personal feelings to a greater extent than is usual in Balint groups.

It was frequently difficult or impossible to understand the origins of the personal pain which was reactivated by some of our patients' personalities. But it was possible to identify the defensive patterns and the kind of patients who provoked them. We were able to identify 'warning lights' – some personal, some of more general application – which informed us that inappropriate defensive behaviour was about to occur. Recognition of these warning signs gave us the opportunity to modify our defences – to open up a little more to our own feelings and those of the patient – before the damage had been done.

In the chapters which follow we describe some of these troubling doctor–patient encounters and show how the doctors' defence mechanisms acted as a barrier to emotional communication. We also give an account of the ways in which the group worked with cases and tried to make sense of them. In the final chapters we make some suggestions about practical ways in which doctors could improve their ability to understand and modify their own defences.

Throughout the book we refer to doctors and not to other health workers. This is merely shorthand. Although our group consisted entirely of doctors we see no reason why the work could not equally have been done by any other professional group involved with consulting with patients. We hope that our story and conclusions will be of interest and of value to all such professional colleagues.

Those of us who took part in the group regarded it as a powerful educational experience which has greatly enhanced our ability to share our patients' feelings in a positive and therapeutic way. It is our hope that those who read this book will find our discoveries not only interesting but capable of transforming their everyday consultations too.

John Salinsky
Paul Sackin
May 2000

About the authors

John Salinsky
General Practitioner
Wembley, Middlesex
VTS Course Organiser
Whittington Hospital, London

Paul Sackin
General Practitioner
Huntingdon, Cambs
VTS Course Organiser
Cambridge

Marie Campkin
General Practitioner
London

Michael Courtenay
Retired General Practitioner
Oxon

Acknowledgements

The authors would like to make it clear that this book belongs to all of the family doctors who worked together in our group over a period of 5 years. They were the people who worked with the patients, presented the cases, discussed the implications and strove together to find meaning in puzzling human experiences. Our debates were vigorous and sometimes painful but always friendly and mutually supportive. The authors' task was to set down the story of the group, to summarise its discoveries and to add some thoughts about future implications for medical education. But without the group and its work there would have been no discoveries and no book.

Our thanks go to our colleagues in the group, Michael Courtenay and Erica Jones (group leaders), Marie Campkin, David Davidson, Peter Graham, Lenka Speight, Heather Suckling and David Watt. Michael Courtenay has written a group leader's preface and he and Marie Campkin have contributed their own valuable chapters to the book. The brief case histories in Chapter 1 were written by the doctors who presented them. Dr Richard Addison provided a good deal of advice and support in the preparation and writing of Chapter 11 and this is greatly appreciated. The course referred to in Chapter 13 was devised and organised by Penny Morris. The late Tom Main's lecture 'Some medical defences against involvement with patients' is reprinted by kind permission of the Council of the Balint Society and of Dr Main's daughter, Dr Jennifer Johns.

Finally, without the patients whose stories are described here, there would have been no book. In order to preserve confidentiality and to avoid any possible hurt, the patients are given fictitious names and some possibly identifiable details are changed without, we hope, altering the essence of the descriptions of the interactions with their doctors. Where we refer in the text to patients and doctors in general we use 'he' or 'him'. We hope readers will accept that this is a convention and not an indication of gender bias by the authors or publishers.

Group leader's preface

Michael Courtenay

The group, whose work generated the research described in this book, began as a response to the realisation that it was a long time since a British Balint group had undertaken a research project. After working for some time on the subject of accidents, group members were becoming dissatisfied, partly because they felt the need to look at a topic which might have a bearing on any case a member might wish to present. This led to the idea of taking up Tom Main's challenge, delivered in the 1978 Balint Memorial Lecture.[1] The fact that the group were mature enough not to throw in the towel after working for 18 months or to leave through pique because of the abandonment of their original idea, speaks volumes for their commitment.

From the leaders' point of view the group was unique in several ways. We were acutely aware of the dedication of the members in regularly giving up half their weekend. We were always conscious that the formation of such a sophisticated group was a rare event and must not, on any account, be wasted. Both leaders were general practitioners, not psychoanalysts, so we felt we had to earn the group's trust every step of the way. Michael Balint had, in the seminal book *The Doctor, His Patient and the Illness*,[2] stated that the leader should attempt to 'merge' with the group. While both leaders had started work in the same group led by him, and we had not noticed that 'merging' was a prominent part of his leadership style, we agreed that, armed with his written intentions, it was entirely appropriate that leadership of the present group must rest on an unwritten contract of special responsibilities among equals.

Under pressure from one or two members of the group, work began to focus more on the doctor contribution in the study of the doctor–patient relationship – that kingpin of Balint work. This was inevitable if the subject under study was doctors' defences. Not surprisingly, there were some initial reservations about this direction of movement in the group. Early presentations appeared to be rather 'cerebral' in nature. They seemed to reflect deliberate attempts to break down the barriers between doctor and (difficult) patient. It was only when a member of the group became so exasperated by a patient that the doctor's emotions could not be completely contained, that the group had the courage to recognise the strength of the need to protect themselves in certain situations. Once that was achieved, steady, if not rapid, progress occurred. Soon, lubricated at times with jokes on the part of both leaders and members, an excitement grew in the group at the prospect of understanding that some defences were the product of events in the doctors' own lives. Far from always being traumatic, such understanding was often both personally liberating and professionally satisfying.

The work was assisted by the discipline of attempting to answer the specific questions hammered out by the group in the quest for understanding the nature of the defences occurring in the reported cases. In this way the intellectual and emotional aspects of the work with the doctor–patient relationship were harnessed to a single vehicle and no longer seen as an inevitable cause of conflict. But this is not to make light of the cost of crossing the divide between personal and professional involvement. In 'classic' Balint work the internal world of the doctor was considered a forbidden area. In his seminars with general practitioners, Michael Balint had sought, with varying success, to establish a boundary between training and treatment. Memories of this produced anxiety in us, as leaders of this research group. If the psychoanalyst leaders had fought shy of moving into the internal worlds of the doctors concerned, were the general practitioner leaders going where angels feared to tread? One important task of a leader had always been to make sure that individual doctors did not come under excessive pressure from their peers. So at what point was the exposure of personal factors in members of the group to be limited? In the event, there was continued pressure from some members to encourage others to greater boldness, often by providing an example. But this was usually contained by the fact that it was explicitly reiterated by the leaders that none of the members were to be forced to expose themselves. Only once did we have to pronounce a moratorium on the discussion of a case, and this was occasioned as much by time constraint as by the possibility of overexposure.

From the leaders' point of view the rewards of the work were enormous. The opportunity to face the challenge of dealing with the effects of the internal worlds of the members in their work with patients opened up a whole new dimension of understanding of what the doctor–patient relationship was about. It was an enormous privilege to face the responsibility of containing possible overexposure by individual members who were prepared to open themselves up in the interest of their work with patients. The heightened level of concentration in the leadership role to accommodate looking at yet another dimension of the group work gave a new level of satisfaction, although it was also extremely exhausting.

Michael and Enid Balint once told me that they thought it needed 5 years for a doctor to reap the full benefit of group work. This was the first time that we, as leaders, had worked with a group that had run the full course. The fact that all the members appeared to emerge unscathed and with deepened insight was a source of great satisfaction to us, not to say relief. There had been many times when the leaders would have loved to have been able to consult their mentor, the late Tom Main. In the event, we came to believe that he would have smiled on our efforts.

References

1   Main T (1978) Some medical defences against involvement with patients. *J Balint Soc.* **7**: 3–11.

2   Balint M (1957) *The Doctor, His Patient and the Illness*. Pitman, London. 2e, 1964; Millennium edition, 2000. Churchill Livingstone, Edinburgh.

1

Morning surgery

Readers may recognise this 'surgery' of patients brought to our seminars by the participating general practitioners:

I looked at the notes before calling Ian in. My heart sank a bit because I saw he had been extensively investigated at a London teaching hospital for myalgic encephalomyelitis (ME). On the other hand, he'd been registered with us for a couple of years and had only been seen twice. I thought maybe he'd got over his ME and he'd just be a quickie today. Ian seemed a pleasant, quiet and intelligent man. His wife came with him and she also seemed very pleasant and reasonable though she did most of the talking. Ian appeared to have a whole string of symptoms and he and his wife were gently insistent that something be done about them. As soon as I tried to understand one symptom, such as the pain in the face, they were on to another and I was quite unable to formulate any plan of action. Twenty minutes passed. They continued to be most 'reasonable' – 'actually, I don't really believe in ME myself, doctor'. By now I felt there was a whole collection of butterflies in my stomach. Were Ian and his wife going to remain in my consulting room all morning? Why couldn't I, a reasonably competent GP with 20 years' experience behind me, get a handle on this consultation?'

• • •

One warm summer afternoon a dapper man of about my own age self-confidently introduced himself to me, shaking my hand. He told me clearly about some persistent upper respiratory symptoms he had suffered recently. They were particularly annoying when he was exercising in a gym. He said he had given up smoking 30–40 a day about 3 months earlier. Like a good doctor I asked whether there was anything else (or was I reading covert signals?). He then simply said that he had 'no joy in life' at the moment. I accepted this, acknowledging it, but dived back into the respiratory symptoms. Hoping to dismiss them and get back to his unhappiness I was shocked to find a wheezy chest, along with his hay fever-like symptoms. Rather than mentioning asthma, I explained his symptoms as hay fever-induced wheeze and suggested an antihistamine. Addressing his 'lack of joy' again, which was not, it seemed, somehow, an urgent problem, I found several things out quickly. He was never married but in a relationship perhaps at a crossroads. I suggested that this might have something to do with the way he felt, gave him the antihistamine prescription, and arranged to see him to continue our talk in 2 weeks' time.

He returned on an afternoon with the thermometer at 33°C, with his tie knot only slightly loosened. The antihistamine had helped a lot. We turned to the other problem and I asked him a lot and found out a little. One of three brothers from Somerset, he did not talk about his emotions to anyone, though he had had a brief private hospitalisation 6 or 7 years before for stress. He had been offered, but declined, ongoing group therapy. He was now working as a self-employed consultant in the City, not earning a great deal, having had a bad work experience/setback a few years before. Yes, he would like to try something like Prozac but felt psychotherapy would be too expensive for him. I felt myself being nominated to care for him. Quite characteristically I offered him a 30-minute appointment in a week or two's time, and uncharacteristically I fished in my drawer for 14 days' worth of Prozac to give him.

• • •

Charlotte has figured largely in my mind since she joined the practice 4 years ago. She came over from Ireland to marry a young man I had actually regarded as possibly homosexual. Anyway, the man's friend moved out, she moved in and was quickly at the surgery with all sorts of 'loud' symptoms starting with sore throats and pains all over and backache and headache and painful periods.... She complained of her pain in such a manic and impulsive way that I was bowled over in the rush of her symptoms. My partners started to demand, 'When are you going to do something about Charlotte?' Eventually, after multiple hospital visits for all her gynaecological problems, she had an ectopic pregnancy and needed a salpingectomy. This only made her immensely more anxious and wound up. She feared she was never going to succeed in having a baby. But soon, to my surprise, she became pregnant and James is now 22 months old. He was 8 weeks premature and everything went wrong in the neonatal period but eventually he was sent home with an apnoea alarm. The trouble is that, nearly 2 years later, James still has his alarm. Charlotte comes rushing in several times a week presenting James's horrific symptoms but he always looks fine to me. She might mention that 'his alarm went off 20 times last night'. She continues to press for 'something to be done'. I agree with her entirely but I suspect that what she wants done is not at all what I think should happen!

• • •

Ruth is a highly skilled and energetic health visitor in her 50s. A while ago we were both involved in the care of two very difficult families and her support and efforts on behalf of the patients were quite remarkable. Sometimes Ruth would ask me a quick question about her own health or request a repeat prescription when I met her at a patient's house. These requests were mildly irritating and were made more difficult by the fact that Ruth often referred to some past consultation which I couldn't remember. My admiration of her work made me feel I should do better.

I got similar feelings when Ruth saw me in the surgery with what looked like thrombophlebitis of her superficial mammary vein. She kept asking me what the problem was and that, 'It can't be serious, can it'? Unfortunately I had an uneasy feeling that it might be serious and felt uncomfortable reassuring her that she didn't have a problem in her *breast* – a half truth, I felt. Then, and at other times, she would make reference to other problems which I simply couldn't remember: 'Why isn't my rash getting better?', 'Might this tiredness be due to my HRT?'. Whenever I hesitated, which was a lot of the time, she would address me by my first name and say something like 'Come on', which I thought was probably teasing but made me feel anxious.

I felt that Ruth would only come to the doctor with 'genuine' illness as she was such a capable woman. When I saw her with the phlebitis I gradually realised that she was actually quite a frequent attender and, a few years before, had had several weeks, if not months, off work with pains in the neck and upper back.

Her 'phlebitis' settled down but she continued to attend frequently with a complaint of tiredness. All blood tests were normal. 'Why am I so tired? Why, WHY?' She was off work and weeks started turning into months. I'm still fond of her and admire her work but I now dread seeing her name on the appointments list.'

• • •

I'd had a reasonably straightforward morning and when it got to

12.15 I wondered about doing my visits and getting off for my half-day. I then noticed that the duty doctor had got very behind with seeing all the extras. There was a young woman in the waiting room who looked vaguely familiar so I thought I'd see her. One more sore throat would hardly delay me that much. Five minutes later I was asking her for the fourth time, 'What can I do for you'? She continued to stare down at her knees. Eventually she started to cry and I handed her the tissues. Suddenly, in between her tears, she started shouting at me. By this time I'd remembered who she was. This pattern of behaviour happens each time she comes, which is surprisingly infrequently. She's always in despair about something, her life really is quite a mess, but it seems that whatever happens it's my fault. Yet she will never see anyone else in the practice.

Eventually, with my own anger mounting, I managed to get out of her that she had lost her job and had no money. However, she was continuing to do some volunteer work with the elderly which, in her state, didn't seem a good idea. She was also continuing with her own counselling. Her counsellor had suggested that she should have some medication. We had an endless discussion about such medication. She started to take detailed notes and said that she would need to discuss it all with her counsellor before she would 'allow' me to prescribe anything. I was getting more and more angry and frustrated, thinking how I could have been enjoying my afternoon off and how I had somehow allowed this woman to 'abuse' me as she had done several times before. By the time we finished, my partner had seen all the other extras and had left the surgery.

• • •

I've known Antonia for a long time. She's a frequent attender and quite demanding. She has hypertension which is quite hard to control, she's prone to depression and she had polio as a child. She has weak legs and walks with crutches though she can push a pram OK. Apparently her father treated her cruelly and blamed her for not being a perfect child, as if the polio was her fault. She knows everything there is to know about polio and the problem now is that she's a single parent with a son who's just over a year old. Somehow she didn't get the expected postnatal depression but now she's really worried that her arms are getting too weak to lift the child. I've examined her several times and her arms don't seem any weaker to me. She's getting into an absolutely dreadful state. She feels she can't bond with the child because she can't hug him properly. It's now getting that she can't cope.

I'd referred her to a London teaching hospital because she'd read about post-polio syndrome and insisted on being referred there, even though her arms hadn't been affected by the polio and I didn't think there was anything wrong with them. They'd investigated her thoroughly and found nothing. She'd also had what was thought to be bilateral carpal tunnel syndrome and she persuaded me to arrange surgery for this at another teaching hospital. Somehow I'd also referred her recently to the local hospital about her elbow pain, which I didn't think was just a simple case of golfer's elbow. These referrals are typical with her. I always feel forced to do exactly what she wants and she makes me feel impotent and constantly manipulated.

Despite her distressed state – she was really going on about how bad her arms were – I suddenly said that, not only wouldn't I expedite her appointment at the local hospital as she wanted, I was going to cancel it. I told her that it was crazy being under three hospitals. This made her really angry. The teaching hospitals were far too far away and she'd walked out of the clinic at one of them. In the middle of this I suddenly had the bizarre thought, 'I haven't done her blood pressure'. As I put the cuff on to do it she started sobbing. She was really in a terribly distressed state. I thought, 'What do I do now? Do I do her blood pressure or not?' I decided to do it. Of course it was massively high. I didn't tell her, just sat down and tried to deal with her distress. Somehow I couldn't deal with it at all and it ended with her standing up and going out crying.

Afterwards she wrote to the health visitor saying that she was very fond of me but I don't listen to her. I was quite wounded by this as I've listened to her like mad and done all sorts of things for her over the years. It's true, though, that I couldn't cope with her at the last consultation. So, I've written to her and asked her to come and see me again. Will I do any better next time?

• • •

I'd seen an unmarried woman of about 60 a couple of times for a sore and itchy vulva. There didn't seem to be any question of anything too serious and I'd prescribed Timodine. A few weeks later she came back and said it had worked well and could she have some more. I agreed, and also let her have some more of her blood pressure medication. She then said, 'Can I ask you about my mother?' It turns out that she lives with her 92-year-old mother who has become preoccupied with anxiety about the electricity bill: 'Have you paid the electricity bill?'; 'Why have you got that fire on?'; 'We can't afford to have all those lights on'. I presumed this was just the case of a demented old woman but somehow it didn't quite seem like that. Alwyn, the patient, then described that her sister would visit and really bully her about the electricity. Both mother and sister would also go on to her if she did some shopping, 'When I go out and come back it's like the Spanish Inquisition'.

I really felt sorry for this woman and found myself, quite uncharacteristically, telling her what to do: why didn't she pay her electricity by direct debit; what about going out more and spending more time on her hobbies. At one point I actually said to her that we were about the same age. I must have been struck with the differences in our lives. My parting shot was, 'If you solved this problem, you'd stop getting your irritation'. I realised I'd been telling her what to do, treating her a bit like a little girl, just as her mother and sister do. But I'm puzzled why they should be so nasty to her.

These were 'real' cases (only altered a little so as to hide their identity) presented to our group. Happily, they did not really all appear in the same surgery session but situations like these will be familiar to those working in primary care. How can GPs cope with such complex problems and such distressed people? If they engage too fully with them they are likely to become overwhelmed and rapidly burnt out. If they keep a 'safe' distance they are unlikely to be able to help the patient much and will become dissatisfied in their work. In the following pages we will be looking at ways in which doctors, and other professionals, might reach a better understanding of their work with such patients. How can they best help them, given the considerable time pressures in the NHS? How can they do useful work without getting too bruised themselves? If 'defences' against complete involvement are necessary, what are the characteristics of these defences? Can we develop 'guidelines' in these areas that might help individual doctors work with particular patients?

2

Setting the scene

'The essential unit of medical practice is the occasion when, in the intimacy of the consulting room or sick room, a person who is ill, or believes himself to be ill, seeks the advice of a doctor whom he trusts. This is a consultation and all else in the practice of medicine derives from it'. This well-known quotation from James Spence[1] perhaps sounds trite nowadays but it helps to remind ourselves of the basis of encounters in general practice: a patient seeking help, a personal doctor who can be trusted and intimate surroundings. Patients certainly seem to believe in the importance of the consultation. For one thing, there are about a million consultations happening every day in general practice in the UK. Patients also seem to welcome the idea of consultations with doctors whom they know and trust and which take place in homely surroundings. There is evidence to suggest that these conditions are considered more important by many patients than the full primary care teams, well-appointed buildings and gleaming computers offered by modern training practices.[2] There is no reason to suggest that patients value a good consultation any less today than they always did. In his uplifting James MacKenzie lecture, John Stevens[3] quotes Emerson, writing in 1838: 'We mark with light in the memory the few interviews we have had, in the dreary years of routine ... with souls that made our souls wiser, that spoke what we thought, that told us what we knew, that gave us leave to be what we inly were'. Yes, patients really do appreciate it if the doctor elicits their ideas, concerns and expectations.[4]

In the education of general practitioners today, great emphasis is rightly placed on the study of the consultation with the aim of teaching young doctors to listen attentively to their patients and to take an interest in them as people. And it isn't just good for patients. Doctors also feel satisfied if they relate positively to their patients. Most of us feel a sense of failure if a consultation has gone wrong and the patient goes away unhappy or resentful. Complaints against doctors are much more likely to occur if patients feel that the doctor was indifferent to their feelings. A diagnosis is more likely to be missed if the doctor is feeling angry or ill-used by the patient. There is some evidence[5,6] that measured health outcomes are favourably influenced by a patient-centred approach to the consultation.

We can help doctors and students to learn the kinds of behaviour in the consultation which will guide them towards being patient-centred.[6] We can teach them to ask open-ended questions and to give the patient time and encouragement to reveal what is on his mind. They can learn to observe non-verbal cues which may reveal hidden emotions. They can learn to foster their capacity for empathy with another human being. Treatment options can be shared so that doctor and patient are more like partners. All these skills are of great value in producing better consultations and improving doctor–patient relationships.

Unfortunately in the modern world life is not as simple as this. There are as many threats to good consultations as there are opportunities for them. These threats come from a variety of sources. Although patients welcome good consultations they can also often get in the way of them, usually for very understandable reasons. For example, overwhelming anxiety in the patient may be manifest as anger and such a patient may seem to make 'unreasonable' demands on the doctor. Often patients' 'wants', perhaps for a quick-fix antibiotic or for a consultation at such an early stage in the illness that diagnosis is very difficult, can mask their 'needs'. Such 'wants' pervade our work as general practitioners just as they do those of other professionals. The father of one of the authors of this book, for example, was a solicitor in a small town. His clients came to him just as distressed as they come to a doctor. The feelings were the same even if the 'presenting problems' – that their neighbour was building an extension that would ruin their view or that they had been accused of theft – were rather different.

Governments have to strike a balance in dealing with the 'wants' and 'needs' of their electorate. Responding to 'wants' may be translated into votes at the next election while concentrating on 'needs' runs the risk of appearing patronising but may win the votes on a longer-term basis. For the government to respond to 'wants' in primary care can cause difficulties. For example, many of today's busy and mobile working population want much better access to health advice than they feel they can get from traditional general practice. Hence the growth, since the mid-1990s, of a variety of alternatives such as NHS Direct, walk-in centres and salaried GPs working in a variety of convenient settings.

These forms of care clearly have many advantages. So do some of the features of modern primary care which have been instigated by doctors. The overwhelming burden of night calls, for example, has been greatly eased by the development of co-operatives. Since the 'Charter' of the mid-1960s there have been incentives for GPs to practise in co-operation with staff so as to share the work and offer a more comprehensive service to patients. Laudable as this 'progress' is in all sorts of ways, it can lead to a less personal service and may well afford fewer opportunities for effective, patient-centred consultations.

Increased accountability and the drive for evidence-based medicine have been features of primary care in recent years, particularly since the time of the 1990 contract for GPs. Doctors have not only had to try and work to high standards, they have had to be seen to be doing so. Again this is a mixed blessing. High standards and an approach based on evidence are manifestly good things but, like any effective medicine, there are side effects. One danger is concentrating on the measurable. For example, records of the HbA1c are undoubtedly an indicator of the quality of care for a patient with diabetes but such measurements fall far short of the true story. They do not say anything about the effect on the patient's life of the diabetes, of his struggles to eat sensibly within a limited budget or about his feelings about having a chronic disease. The whole audit process (and now clinical governance) is predicated on agreeing criteria and standards of care and measuring performance in relation to those standards.[7] It is so much easier to set standards that are readily measurable and credibility is enhanced if those standards relate to clear-cut recent evidence.

These priorities for general practice may well reflect those of our society. Yet individual patients (and that includes all of us) yearn for the personal consultation and for those difficult-to-measure criteria such as warmth, understanding and empathy.

Even if these 'external' factors mitigating against effective consultations can be overcome, there are still difficulties. In 1957, Michael Balint[8] wrote: 'Why does it happen so often that, in spite of earnest efforts on both sides, the relationship between patient and doctor is unsatisfactory and even unhappy?' Forty years later we are still some way from resolving this problem, despite even greater efforts. It is a common experience that consultations still go wrong and relationships deteriorate. This is not because we do not know how to behave but because there are occasions when we seem unable to behave appropriately. We find that without wanting it to happen, or even being aware of how it happened, a consultation has gone badly wrong.

Why does it happen? The clue seems to lie in the disruptive emotions which are generated in both doctor and patient. One or other or both will be feeling angry, hurt, indignant, depressed or anxious; or perhaps just self-righteous. If we are honest with ourselves and reflect on what has happened, we realise that we have been surprised by some strong emotions which we hadn't anticipated. There has been a failure of self-awareness. Some very powerful (unconscious) force seems to have been blocking our ability to use our consultation skills and our capacity for empathy. It is our hypothesis in this book that this powerful force is a defence mechanism which protects doctors from being over-whelmed and seriously disabled by too much exposure to the distress of their patients. As doctors, we are trained from an early age to defend ourselves against too much feeling. We enter the dissecting room at the age of 18, when we are little more than chil-dren. We are unceremoniously thrust into contact with grotesque and chilly corpses when most of us have only experienced the human form as something alive and warm. We soon learn to make jokes about it and shrug off the presence of death. How else could we concentrate on learning our anatomy? Soon afterwards we are in the wards where the people are still warm but many are seriously ill. They and their families may be grievously distressed and in pain. We learn to 'cope' with this by shutting ourselves off from the feelings. Jokes and camaraderie are a great help. The suffering can become distanced and unreal. The patient in bed 3 is just 'the cerebrovascular accident (CVA)' or 'the hysterectomy'. We are learning to be 'professionals'.

We may come to believe that it is possible and desirable to develop a 'professional self' who handles all our business activities and is unaffected by human emotions. Meanwhile the 'personal self' inhabits a different space inside us and is never affected by the emotions of our patients. It may just be possible to sustain this illusion in some specialties – but not in general practice. Our work brings us too close to our patients' personalities and emotions for this to be sustainable. From time to time our patients' distress resonates with something painful in our personal history. We soon realise that the professional self is only a specialised part of the personal self. And the personal self remains quite vulnerable to feelings aroused during our professional activities. Some defences are clearly necessary to enable us to survive in the job. When one person cries in the surgery it is quite affecting for a sensitive doctor. When several people do it we would be devastated if we were not able to distance ourselves to some extent from the cumulative distress.

The problem is that the defensive withdrawal may be too sudden and too abrupt. We need to be able to share our patients' feelings to some extent, including the sad and angry ones, if we are to achieve some measure of understanding of what they are going through and what they need from us emotionally. If our defences are too rigid, if we are unable to take a few risks with our feelings, then we find ourselves professionally disabled in a different way. To give an obvious example, we may miss a diagnosis of depression. We may be so cut off from communicating with the patient that we miss other important diagnoses as well. We may be unable to provide help and support when they are needed because we are so frosty and reserved.

We need to protect ourselves in order to survive. But we also need to be able to share painful feelings when it is helpful to do so and not too dangerous. How can we get the balance right?

This book describes the work of a group of experienced family doctors who tried to explore this problem and find some answers to it. Our interest was inspired by a thought-provoking lecture given to the Balint Society in 1978, and subsequently published.[9] The lecture is reproduced here as an Appendix. It was given by Tom Main, a distinguished psychoanalyst, who worked with Michael Balint and shared his interest in the doctor–patient relationship in primary care. Main argued that family doctors employed all sorts of largely unconscious defences to protect themselves from an emotional engagement with the patient which might be devastating. However, the defences are often out of proportion to the need and prevent the doctor from being able to share the patient's feelings in a way which is helpful and therapeutic. Main suggested that, by examining these defences and the emotions which give rise to them, doctors in a Balint seminar might be able to avoid automatic, unthinking defences actuated by unconscious fears. When defences were really necessary for the doctor's protection they would be consciously and deliberately employed. We were excited and enthusiastic about this challenge and decided to adopt it as our research project. But we would like to begin by describing a few examples of 'doctors' defences' as they operate in the everyday surgery consultation.

References

1   Spence J (1960) *The Purpose and Practice of Medicine.* Oxford University Press, Oxford.

2   Baker R (1997) Will the future GP remain a personal doctor? *Br J Gen Pract.* **47**: 821–3.

3   Stevens J (1974) Brief encounter. *J Roy Coll Gen Pract.* **24**: 5–22.

4   Pendleton, D, Schofield T, Tate P, Havelock P (1984) *The Consultation: an approach to learning and teaching.* Oxford University Press, Oxford.

5   Stewart M, Belle Brown J, Wayne Weston W *et al.* (1995)

Patient-centred Medicine: transforming the clinical method. Sage Publications, Thousand Oaks, CA.

6   Silverman J, Kurtz S, Draper J (1998) *Skills for Communicating with Patients.* Radcliffe Medical Press, Oxford.

7   Samuel O, Sackin P, Sibbald B (1993) *Counting on Quality.* Royal College of General Practitioners, Exeter.

8   Balint M (1957) *The Doctor, His Patient and the Illness.* Pitman, London. 2e, 1964; Millennium edition, 2000. Churchill Livingstone, Edinburgh.

9   Main T (1978) Some medical defences against involvement with patients. *J Balint Soc.* **7**: 3–11.

3

Some doctors and their defences

The disintegrating hearing aid

One of the GPs in our group presented the following case:

I knew she would be trouble before I even set eyes on her. I was told by the receptionist that a 90-year-old lady had just been struck off the list of a neighbouring practice and was looking for a new doctor to register with. I know the doctors in her old practice very well and I felt sure they wouldn't refuse to go on looking after an elderly lady unless she had really given them a hard time. You don't feel very happy about someone who comes with that sort of introduction but I agreed to talk to her to see how the first interview went before I decided. And so she came in, a very fit and active-looking 90-year-old lady, but she had a swelling under her jaw. She had just had some dental work done and it wasn't quite clear whether this lump was a gland resulting from a tooth infection or from something else altogether. Before I could give that much thought she moved on to tell me about all sorts of other problems that she had. She had a little list of the various specialists I would need to contact about her heart and her arthritis and her chronic blood disorder. It soon became apparent that her relationships with her specialists were fairly stormy. She had dismissed one cardiologist because he had been rude to her and the other one was far from satisfactory – so could I recommend a third one? There were also problems with her hearing and at that point she said would I look in her ears to see if there was any wax there?

Before I could stop her she had removed both her hearing aids, one of which instantly fell apart into about six pieces which rolled all over my desk. And of course once she had removed them she could no longer hear me. She tried to put the intact one back again and couldn't, and I tried to reassemble the one that had fallen apart – and couldn't – and I started to panic. I think panic is the only word to describe it really. I thought, I just can't cope with this. There were mad thoughts in my mind like, 'I'm going to be sitting here for ever playing with bits of hearing aid and shouting at this terrible old woman who can't hear me and I shall have to spend hours writing stupid letters to consultants for her. It will be like this all the time from now on. No wonder the other doctor sacked her and why should I have to suffer this instead of him?' Then I heard her saying: 'Can I see you every time I come? What I like is to have one doctor I can go to all the time. I don't like having to see different ones. I got on very well with Dr X until he suddenly said I had to leave his practice. I don't know what got into him when he said that'. I knew. I started to become very defensive. I heard myself giving a little speech about how we were a group practice and it was impossible to see one doctor all the time. (In fact this is quite untrue. We pride ourselves on the way we follow up our patients personally.) And then I began to say even worse things: that I didn't think it was a good idea for her to join our practice; we weren't the sort of practice she was looking for and she would do much better to try somewhere else and for God's sake get those bits of hearing aid off my desk and get out of here. I was really fuming and shaking by that stage, totally out of control. I don't know if she could hear me but she got the message, perhaps she read my body language. She got up, took her bits and pieces and went off shaking her head . . .

We have to wonder why this encounter gave rise to such bad behaviour on the part of the doctor. GPs (including this doctor) are normally friendly, open and interested in patients as people. They are generally patient, considerate, caring professionals who are kind to old ladies. You may be shocked to hear that an experienced GP, highly regarded by his colleagues and many of his patients, could so forget himself. How did this patient manage to reduce the doctor to a state of panic (his own phrase) and professional disintegration? What made him come to pieces in the same way as the offending hearing aid? The answer might be that the old lady did it. But how can a fragile old lady have such a devastating effect on an experienced practitioner? We might be reminded of the classic Ealing comedy film *The Ladykillers*, in which another old lady (just as single-minded) reduces Alec Guinness's team of hardened professional criminals to despair and mutual destruction. Could something similar be operating here? Is it really possible for an innocent old lady to be responsible for such a startling deterioration in a doctor's behaviour?

Anyone familiar with general practice will recognise a number of elements in the situation which are likely to distress and possibly unbalance a family doctor. First of all, the patient is preceded by the dread warning – removed from the list of another doctor. She must have committed terrible acts in order to have evoked the supreme sanction. When she appears her presentation is long and meandering, perhaps when the doctor was already feeling pressed for time. Then she makes demands on him which he finds quite unreasonable. Her medical history is already unnecessarily complicated and he will be expected to familiarise himself with the details, like a barrister learning a brief. He will have to act as her intermediary with her consultants who are probably already fed up with her for wasting their time. He is expected to mend her hearing aid, a task both undignified and beyond his competence. Finally, having spread her disintegration all over his desk, she is expecting him to be her personal doctor, with no one to share the responsibility. An endless perspective of similar consultations opens up before him. He will be enslaved for ever to the demented demands of this imperious and self-absorbed old person. There may be other things about her that stir up personal, private anxieties of which he is unconscious or only partly conscious. Whatever the contributory causes, something seems to have snapped inside him. He has feelings he described as panic and madness. His customary behaviour is totally changed. It is as if a massive armour-plated steel door had descended with lightning speed, sealing off the doctor's normal warm, affable professional self. Instead of being treated with consideration and respect, the patient is now treated with lack of understanding, coldness, hostility and even rudeness.

Happily, this is not the end of the story. The doctor continued his account as follows:

As soon as she left the room I began to have feelings of remorse and so I followed her. I didn't know where she was going. When I caught up with her she had got as far as the receptionist and the bits of hearing aid were now spread on her counter. The receptionist was just sitting there with her arms folded and I could see from her expression that she was being defensive too. So I appealed to one of the other receptionists, whom I thought would be more practical, and asked her if she could help put the hearing aid together. She said she would have a go at it and I said to the patient, 'This lady will help you with the hearing aid and after that I will see you again'. And the old lady said, 'No, no I don't think I will after what you said. I have my pride, you know'. So I said, 'Look, I'm sorry about that. Let's get your hearing aid together so you can hear me and then let's try again'. So she agreed. The receptionist very cleverly reassembled the hearing aid and she came back with both aids in place, and the curious thing is that, having gone out of control, gone quite mad for a bit, I was then able to be much more in control and felt much better about the whole thing. We had quite a reasonable conversation. I undertook to contact the cardiologist and the haematologist and see her again after she had been to the dentist. So she made another appointment and went home, leaving her glasses behind. I actually delivered the glasses to her house myself because I felt so bad about the whole business.

When the old lady left the room clutching her dignity and her fragments of hearing aid the doctor suddenly came to his senses. The protective steel door retracted, the doctor's humanity emerged blinking into the sunlight and he tried to put things right. He now realised that his defences had been out of all proportion to the 'threat' which had been facing him. In reality he had been quite safe all the time. The hearing aid could be mended with a little assistance. There might be a need for some restraining influence in the matter of multiple consultant opinions but this could be managed by negotiation between two fairly reasonable human beings. In reality, the old lady was not a monster threatening his way of life but a fellow creature who needed his help.

As a result of his prompt recovery and the undoing of his unnecessary defences, the doctor was able to retrieve the immediate situation. In subsequent reports to the group he told us that he had had two more quite amicable consultations with the old lady. But after that she had attached herself to one of his female partners and chosen her as her regular doctor. Although our doctor was relieved that someone else had now taken on this difficult patient, his professional pride was also a little hurt by her 'defection'.

During the subsequent discussion in the group, the doctor revealed that his own mother, who was in her 90s, was also profoundly deaf and refused even to consider wearing a hearing aid. He had to shout to make himself heard when he was with her and often felt very angry with her. Members of the group wondered if other doctors would also have felt angry with this lady and pointed out that there was evidence that they would. One GP had fired her and at least one specialist had been rude to her! Nevertheless, the doctor felt that her deafness had a special meaning for him and that some of the feelings she induced in him really belonged to his relationship with his mother.

In our group meetings we heard many other stories about doctors who felt threatened in various ways and who also reacted with instant defensive mechanisms. Sometimes, instead of becoming overtly hostile, the doctor would take shelter behind a screen of polite and superficially correct behaviour which insulated him from any contact with the patient's feelings. A doctor might invoke all sorts of regulations and 'practice policies' which effectively deny the patient what he really wants.

Another case from our group will illustrate this sort of reaction:

'I'd like some sleeping tablets'

The patient was a 30-year-old man, tall, slim and dressed in black. The doctor found his face familiar but couldn't remember where or when she had seen him before. She said, 'How can I help you?'

and he said, 'I'd like some sleeping tablets'. The doctor told us, 'I was quite aware of my allergy to that'. They looked at each other in silence for a few minutes, the doctor being determined not to be the first to break the silence. The patient then repeated his request and the doctor thought, 'This is not going to be a nice consultation'. She said to him, 'Well, tell me about it ...', but our impression was that this was not said in a very inviting way. While the patient tried to decide whether to share his innermost thoughts or keep them to himself, the doctor glanced at his notes (which were quite thin) and found that he had previously asked her for sleeping tablets several years ago and they must have had a similar collision. Doctor and patient then had a very scratchy and uncomfortable conversation. The patient revealed that he had previously been promised a referral to a counsellor for help with his drinking. He had great difficulty in sleeping and drank heavily at night to try to get to sleep. However, he also believed that the sleeping difficulty was inherited because his father never needed much sleep and he himself could manage perfectly well on 3 or 4 hours. This prompted the doctor to enquire rather ironically whether 'after drinking all that alcohol you actually fall asleep or do you spend those 3 hours of the night just sitting there drinking and then go to bed and get your 3 hours' sleep?'

During the course of the interview, the patient revealed a number of other things about his life. He worked as an engineer but also had a small practice as a counsellor. He had been in therapy himself for many years and had been feeling depressed because of a breakdown in his relationship with a long-standing partner. The doctor seemed to have extracted all this information in a series of sudden jerks, rather like pulling teeth. She normally has a very warm, sympathetic approach to her patients but with this patient, on this occasion, her defences had replaced her humanity with an icy, slightly scornful formality. In the end, she gave him a piece of paper referring him to the local alcohol counselling service because she had decided that his self-confessed extremely high alcohol intake was the problem which needed addressing first. 'And he left and he was miserable and I was miserable because I was bored. I thought, "Well, I don't really need this. If somebody doesn't want my advice, why does he come? There should be a notice in the waiting room, 'Dr A doesn't prescribe sleepers'".'

The request (demand?) for sleeping tablets as an opening gambit seems to have activated a hair-trigger defence mechanism in a doctor who is 'allergic' to sleeping tablets. The doctor later noted that she might also have a tendency to be 'allergic' to patients who described themselves as 'counsellors' or 'psychotherapists'. As in the case of the lady with the hearing aid, the defences were brought into play instantly and automatically before the doctor had time to realise what was happening. Another analogy might be the way the air bag in a modern car will open rapidly and instantly to protect the driver's chest from impact with the steering wheel – perhaps before the driver has even realised that there is going to be a collision. Events happen with frightening speed in car crashes and the air bag mechanism has to work instantly. But collisions between doctor and patients happen more slowly. It should be possible to anticipate them and modify our defences if they seem to be out of proportion to the threat. If only this doctor had been able to give herself time to think: 'This patient is asking for sleeping tablets which I never prescribe. I am going to feel uncomfortable about this but maybe I can set that aside for the moment and listen to his story, try to see things from his point of view as I normally do with any other troubled person who comes to see me. I feel that he has come here just to abuse me but it probably does not feel like that to him.'

In this example, the patient seems to have committed a succession of acts which made the doctor feel more and more cold towards him. She felt some antipathy for him right from the outset when he marched into the consulting room ahead of her. Then she remembered him from a previous consultation which was also slightly disturbing. His next 'mistake' was to ask for sleeping tablets from a doctor who makes no exceptions to her ban on prescribing them. She asked him to 'tell me about it' but without her usual enthusiasm. Instead of being interested, she felt bored. While he was talking she flicked through his (thin) folder and found a previous encounter in her own handwriting, 8 years earlier, in which he had also asked for sleeping tablets. His bland admissions about his heavy drinking did nothing to help his case but the final factor in sealing the doctor's defences tightly was his description of himself as 'a behavioural psychotherapist'.

In the discussion that followed, we puzzled over the ways in which the patient's behaviour had disturbed and affronted the doctor. She had had no personal problems with sleeping tablets and her policy of not prescribing them was purely professional in origin. The rest of us agreed with this policy although we were not all able to hold the line so firmly. We all felt a little uneasy about 'psychotherapists' as patients, perhaps because they made us feel challenged by someone who might have greater therapeutic skills. Our presenting doctor felt particularly cool towards people who described themselves as psychotherapists and had set themselves up in practice without proper supervision and training. The experience of a member of her own family with an unsatisfactory therapist had reinforced this negative feeling. Another point which came out in the discussion was that there had been no opportunity for 'negotiation'. Doctor and patient were not able to discuss calmly why one felt desperately in need of sleeping tablets and the other believed strongly that they should be avoided. Towards the end of the discussion, the doctor said that she did not like the idea that she had been 'a horrible person' to this patient and that perhaps she needed to rethink her attitude towards him.

It seems that our defences have some intrinsic tendency to act before we are scarcely even aware of a threat. Slowing the process down seems to be immensely difficult, even though we know intellectually that the consequences would be beneficial. The speed of operation, quicker than conscious thought, seems to be one of the main obstacles to our efforts to understand and control our defences. And they need controlling because so often they are inappropriately massive and damaging to our professional effectiveness.

We also heard stories involving a rather different kind of defence which seems to be trying to protect both doctor and patient. On these occasions the doctor seems to be shielding the patient from painful feelings which the doctor may find almost intolerable himself. The following case is a good example:

A lump in the breast

The patient was a 46-year-old woman whom the doctor had known for many years. She came to the surgery quite rarely and usually only for routine procedures such as cervical smears. But now she had come in some distress because she had found a lump in her breast. Our doctor saw her in the afternoon surgery but she had already been seen by a locum doctor the same morning and referred to a breast clinic (the wrong one, as it turned out). She said, 'I know I was here this morning but I'm beside myself. Would you mind having a look as well'? The doctor examined her and found a small lump just over 1 cm long and very mobile. 'It really felt like a fibroadenoma (a totally benign tumour) and I said, "Well, you know one can never tell but I have to say I can't find any worrying features". And the patient said, "Well, how long will I have to wait?" and I said, "Well, I'll try and get you an urgent appointment. I'll fax the letter through because I can see you're terribly anxious"'. The doctor did so but when the patient did get an appointment a week later it was for a date a month in the future. The doctor was furious, telephoned the clinic and discovered that there had been a mistake. This was rapidly rectified and the patient was given an appointment for the following morning. After the clinic visit the consultant telephoned the GP and told her that the tumour was a cancer. The needle biopsy had been positive and there was an enlarged node in the axilla. The patient and her husband had both been very shocked at the news and both had fainted! The doctor also felt devastated because she had been convinced that the tumour was benign and had been very reassuring. However, when the patient came to see her the following week (2 weeks after the initial examination) the lump was much more irregular with skin tethering. At first the patient said, 'I know I'm going to die and what will happen to my children and does it make any difference if I have any treatment?' She cried quite a lot but eventually calmed down enough to discuss the probable treatment options and what she and her husband should tell their two daughters.

When the group discussed this case, there was a general feeling that the doctor felt so protective about this nice patient who never gave any trouble, that she had unconsciously set up a defence against admitting even to herself that the lump might well be malignant. The doctor found this idea that she had been overprotective hard to accept because at the first consultation the lump had looked so innocent. The group also noted that despite her lack of anxiety about the pathology of the lump, she had been very angry with the hospital when there was a mix up over the appointment and she made sure that the patient was seen as early as possible. The doctor reasoned that she had had problems with 'urgent' appointments at the clinic before and she wanted to make sure that they were seeing everyone with any kind of breast lump as soon as possible. The group members continued to feel that the doctor's own dread of really bad news for this particular patient had made her deny the possibility to herself and the patient – while at the same time moving heaven and earth to get her assessed quickly.

Would the doctor have behaved differently if she had been aware of her defences? She might have spent time with the patient dealing with her fears in anticipation of a possible diagnosis of cancer, although it is questionable whether the patient would have wanted this at that stage. When reviewing the case at a later date the group also discussed whether this doctor was more upset by the diagnosis of breast cancer in a woman of 46 than other doctors might have been. We agreed that we all felt seriously disturbed by breast cancer, the men as well as the women. The doctor herself now agreed that she might have been influenced by defensive processes. She had no personal or family history of breast cancer or any reason to be more upset by it than the rest of us. But she felt that she had picked up very strongly the patient's terror of breast cancer at the first interview. She reminded us that when the patient and her husband were told the grim news by the consultant, they both fainted. In this case it would be hard to argue that the doctor's defences had any adverse effect on the outcome. The patient was referred very speedily, perhaps because the doctor shared the patient's fear of the worst.

The 'personal self' and the 'professional self'

These defences all have in common the need to protect the doctor's personal-feeling self from what seem to be intolerable pain, grief, anxiety or depression. Some sort of defence system is absolutely necessary for us if we are not to be overwhelmed by the pain and anguish of all those people who come to us for help and want us to share their feelings. Without some protection in the form of the ability to distance ourselves, we would not be able to survive professionally. But too much fear can lead to defences which are out of proportion to the need. As students we were taught, by example if not by instruction, that a doctor must have a 'professional self' who wears a crisply starched white coat and is able to perceive everything with total objectivity. He listens courteously to the patient's 'history' and extracts from it (with the aid of questions) the necessary data to make a diagnosis. If the history is related with tears and a catch in the voice, if the tale it tells is of terrible suffering, the professional self will, if it seems relevant, register these facts and make use of them in his diagnosis but he does not feel them personally. He is like the doctor in a short story by Ernest Hemingway called *Indian Camp*.[1] In this story, a doctor is about to perform a caesarean section on a native American woman in obstructed labour, without using an anaesthetic. When his little son asks him what he is going to do about the woman's screams, the doctor replies: '... her screams are not important. I don't hear them because they are not important'.

Now we family doctors know that you cannot really practise medicine like that. In addition to the professional self there is a personal self whom we ignore at our peril (and that of the patient). It is through our personal self that we make contact with the patient as one human being with another. If we try to shut the personal self away when we see our patients they are deprived of the empathy and warmth that enables them to feel that they have been truly heard and that they are cared for. There is some objective evidence that this enhances the rate of healing of traumatised tissues. It is certainly widely recognised that good communication skills and an effective doctor–patient relationship are the essential foundations of good medical care. And even if it were not so, medicine would be a heartless, cruel and unnatural occupation for human beings to engage in if we never involved our own feelings. Now we must recognise that the personal self is exposed to considerable dangers when we allow it into the consulting room, as Tom Main[2] showed in the paper which sparked off our research project. The physical, mental and spiritual suffering of our patients can be intolerable if we expose our professional selves to the fiery heat of their pain without any protection. Hence, the need for defences. But if we try to protect the personal self by denying it any access to the battle zone we deprive the patients and ourselves of the mixture of objectivity and subjectivity which seems to be necessary for good personal doctoring. Enid Balint has described in *While I'm Here, Doctor*,[3] the way in which we as clinicians allow ourselves to approach closely, and identify with, a patient's feelings, to experience empathically something of their emotional state – and then step back again. By stepping back a little we can then examine the feelings we have experienced and consider what they mean. In this way we can also avoid being totally immersed in the patient's feelings and drowning before we can rescue them. But judging the distance and the timing between risky engagement and safe tactical withdrawal is not easy. Stay too close and you lose objective judgement and the ability to intervene effectively. Do not go near at all and you are safe, but the personal self never has a chance to make its vital contribution.

Sometimes the doctor's sympathy is aroused and he approaches the patient's feeling self more closely. Then, unexpectedly, the doctor experiences a sudden threat, a whiff of danger which makes him withdraw again hurriedly behind his defences. The personal self has peeped out tentatively and then disappeared again leaving only the imperturbable facade of the professional self. In our group, we developed the metaphor of the doctor as a kind of 'amoeba' in order to describe the dynamics of this process.

If our sketchy memories of school biology are correct, the amoeba puts out a pseudopodium when attracted by an external object which might be suitable for ingestion. Protoplasm from the main body of the amoeba's cell flows out into the pseudopodium. The amoeba transfers its substance towards the object, touches it and may then engulf it. If it then experiences a noxious chemical substance, the pseudopodium is quickly withdrawn and the protoplasm flows back towards the centre so that the amoeba resumes a more spherical shape. We likened the doctor's personal self to the inner protoplasm which flows easily into the professional pseudopodium extended towards the patient – only to be withdrawn again quickly when danger threatens. This image of the amoeba allowed us to see the personal 'protoplasm' as an essential substance which is a natural part of the professional process extended towards the patient. A good doctor–patient relationship needs the involvement of the personal self. At the same time we must protect our personal selves if we are to maintain our own good health and survive to be available for the next patient and the one after that.

How can we learn to understand and have some control over the powerful defence mechanisms which we have seen in action in the case studies in this chapter? We have seen that they operate with alarming swiftness in response to danger signals of which we are barely conscious. We do not wish to disable our defences entirely because they will always be needed. However, it would seem that the more massive defences, those involving total withdrawal and seclusion of the personal self, are only needed in extreme circumstances. More often, when the alarm goes off, the danger is more apparent than real. The defences could be considerably scaled down if not switched off completely. But how can we tell? Is it possible to be forewarned of a defensive shutdown or the imminent firing of a retaliatory missile before the process is irreversible? During the Cold War the American and Soviet presidents had a 'hot line' on which they could talk to each other immediately if either of their defence systems had detected a threat which might be a false alarm. Do we have a hot line to our patients? Can we communicate with our own defence systems? Is there at least a red light which will flash and warn us that war is about to break out? We obviously need to study our defences and the ways in which they are activated. In the next chapter we describe how our group set about trying to gain a better understanding of these processes.

References

1   Hemingway E (1924) Indian camp. In: *The First Forty-nine Stories* (published 1993). Arrow Books, London.

2   Main T (1978) Some medical defences against emotional involvement with patients. *J Balint Soc.* **7**: 3–11.

3   Balint E (1987). In: A Elder, O Samuel (eds), *While I'm Here, Doctor*. Routledge, London.

4

The work of the group

The members of our research group met regularly for several years to explore the problem of doctors' emotional defences and the ways in which, if inappropriate, these defences can impair the consultation process and the doctor–patient relationship. Many research studies on the psychosocial aspects of medicine have used quantitative methods. While these methods provide 'hard' data, they are not as reliable as the data from physical or even biological research. A more serious objection is that numbers cannot always provide answers to the more interesting questions about human behaviour. We may be able to determine how many doctors behave in a particular way but we learn nothing about what motivates them or the ways in which they differ as individuals. For this sort of enquiry a different approach is needed and in recent years it has increasingly been provided by qualitative research.[1] While not providing information with the same precision, qualitative methods are able to slip into the spaces in between 'the known facts' and find answers to questions beginning 'why' and 'how' rather than 'what' or 'how many'. They are also able to discover which questions need to be asked.

Modern qualitative research techniques often involve tape-recorded semi-structured interviews and the analysis of discussions in focus groups. An example of this kind of enquiry will be found in Chapter 11 of this book. For over 40 years, general practice has had its own qualitative research instrument in the form of the case discussion group pioneered by Michael Balint in London. Balint's classic work, *The Doctor, His Patient and the Illness*,[2] has had an enormous influence on the development of general practice in Britain and many other countries. The book documented the work of a group of GPs led by Michael Balint and described by him as taking part in 'research-cum-training' seminars. Since then Balint seminars have played an important part in education for family medicine in many countries. Their use in research has been less common, perhaps because their potential for qualitative research is only just becoming fully recognised. Richard Addison, a social scientist and psychologist, has written about hermeneutic research and has also worked with Balint groups. He has drawn attention to a number of close parallels between Balint work and hermeneutic methods of qualitative research.[3] Both methods are engaged in a search for meaning and understanding by means of entering the situation or world which is being examined and trying to understand it experientially. Puzzles and contradictions are unearthed and background assumptions, including those of the investigator, are examined. Further interpretations are then made in the light of reflection and further experience. The Balint group, according to Addison, may be seen as 'a community of shared experience' whose members are using hermeneutic methods to help each other in the carrying out of meaningful work, in this case their caring for and 'connectedness' with their patients.

In Britain, most Balint seminars continue to be run in the format established by Michael Balint. A group of about 6 to 12 GPs meet for one and a half hours, traditionally on a weekly basis. Where possible they are co-led by a GP and by a psychotherapist. Balint's opening was invariably, 'Who has a case?' After a pause of variable length, a case or two is 'offered'. Cases are usually accounts of patients who have been disturbing the doctor in some way. Usually two new cases are discussed in each session and some time is also devoted to follow-up reports. A key feature of the groups is that the presenter does not bring notes. What he or she forgets and any hesitations in the presentation are not to be criticised. Instead, they are likely to reflect the relationship between the doctor and the patient which is the focus of the discussion. Once the doctor has finished the presentation the leader allows the inevitable questioning of the presenter to establish matters of fact. After that it is important to keep such interrogation to a minimum. The way the group reacts emotionally to the case and the difficulties members encounter with the work are likely to reflect what is happening between the doctor and the patient. Group members need to work creatively to explore and attempt to understand the doctor–patient relationship. This increased understanding empowers the presenting doctor to move forward. Other group members should also gain insight which will help them with their own patients.

Our method of working was based very much on this model. For practical reasons we met for a whole day at a time, approximately five times per year. We were led by Michael Courtenay and Erica Jones, two retired GPs with enormous experience of leading Balint groups both for training and research. All our discussions were audio-recorded and most of them were transcribed. After we had been meeting together for some time researching another subject (and had become a well-established and 'safe' group) we decided that it might be more fruitful to turn our attention to doctors' defences and to take up some of the challenges laid down by Tom Main and described in Chapter 2.

We agreed to proceed as follows:

1   Group members would present cases which were concerning them in some way, making them uncertain as to how to proceed. While no cases would be excluded if they were troubling the doctor, the group would be particularly interested in examples of 'over-defensive' behaviour which had apparently prevented the doctor from listening with empathy and behaving effectively in a professional capacity.

2   At the end of each presentation and discussion formal questions would be asked with reference to possible defence mechanisms.

3   At the beginning of each subsequent meeting, after perusal of the transcript of the last meeting, there would be a review (and

possible follow-up) of each case in order to try and ascertain how the group might have helped the doctor more and to re-examine what defence mechanisms might have been involved.

We felt that this approach was important to ensure safety because, in looking at defences, it might only be possible to make sense of the doctor–patient relationship by allowing certain personal experiences of group members to emerge. This would appear to break the classical Balint dictum that only professional issues should be discussed. Yet it was becoming clear to us that, to paraphrase Balint, a considerable, though limited, change in our method of working was necessary if we were to rise to Tom Main's challenge. We also felt that shifting the spectrum of the doctor–patient relationship a little towards the doctor end might be a model that would appeal to our stressed and distressed colleagues in general practice. Yet we were all clear that any personal revelations were in the interests of helping us to understand the doctor–patient relationship and furthering our research on doctors' defences. It would be a useful side effect if members felt supported by their colleagues in the group (which we were). But the group was to be no more a therapy group than any other Balint group. This more humanistic approach to Balint work seems to be similar to that in many groups in Germany[5] and may be a factor in their relative popularity there.

The use of formal questions seemed essential for us to focus on the defence mechanisms. The final version of the questions took quite some time to evolve. We needed to discuss some cases first and develop enough safety in the group for participants to feel confident about making personal revelations. Eventually the questions we agreed were as follows.

- What was the nature of the defence(s)?

- What was it about the patient that upset the doctor?

- Would this have upset *other* doctors?

- If the doctor had been aware of the *nature* of the upset at the time, what might have happened?

- How was the outcome affected?

We spent a lot of time, sometimes with considerable heat, in discussing the exact wording of the questions. The most anguished debate was over the word 'upset'. Perhaps it sounds a bit dramatic. The doctor did not *have* to be distressed to present the case. 'Puzzled', 'confused' and 'pressured' were some alternative words we considered at length. However, we couldn't think of a better word and if we use the word 'upset' literally – implying some instability in the doctor's equilibrium – we think it works well to convey our meaning. At the centre of our research was the issue of the effect of patients on particular doctors. Clearly, some patients, such as violent ones or those with grave illnesses, will distress most doctors. Our interest was in trying to prevent inappropriate and unconscious defences and so we were keen in our research to highlight cases that seemed to cause an 'upset' to the particular presenting doctor. The questions seemed the best way of focusing our thinking on identifying participants' defences and looking at what could be done to make them more conscious and appropriate.

When it came to discussing either the transcript of the initial discussion or follow-up consultations we had to use slightly different questions. This was the final version we arrived at for these.

• Does (a) the discussion of the transcript or (b) the discussion of follow-up consultation(s) throw new light on any defence mechanisms?

• Are any fresh defence mechanisms discernible at the follow-up consultation(s)?

• At what point did the doctor gain insight into the nature of the defences(s)?

• How have subsequent encounters been affected by the insight and comments of the group?

Somewhat to our surprise, once we had arrived at an agreed version of the questions, it became easier for participants to understand and reveal their defences. This was rarely possible immediately after presenting the case. It usually occurred after discussing the transcript of the initial discussion, often during the formal stage of the group's work when we tried to answer each question in turn.

Sometimes the discussion of follow-up consultations gave important new insights into the doctor–patient relationship and the nature of the defences. Group members were encouraged to present follow-ups as in any Balint group. In addition, during the third year of the group's work, we gave an opportunity to each doctor to go briefly over all their cases again. This was partly to satisfy the curiosity of the other group members. From the research point of view, we saw it as important to review any changes in the defence mechanisms and to see whether the group discussions had been helpful to the presenting doctor.

The group therefore functioned on a number of different planes. It was an 'ordinary' Balint group, discussing cases that were troubling the presenting doctors. It also looked at some personal issues in greater depth than is usually the case, at least in Britain. At the same time there was a definite structure to the proceedings. We asked formal questions about the doctors' defences. We revisited these questions when discussing the transcript of each session and when discussing follow-up consultations.

Towards the end of the group's work we looked briefly at all the cases again, trying to see if any patterns were emerging. In addition to this work, we spent time discussing our presentation to the International Balint Congress in Oxford in September 1998,[6] and this process gave us some new insights into our work. There was also a lot of written material. After each session Michael Courtenay sent all group members a brief summary of each case discussion which helped jog our memories and crystallise our thoughts before the arrival of the full transcript. Finally, at various times, Michael Courtenay and some other members of the group circulated for discussion their thoughts on how our work was progressing and what insights they saw developing. We hope that the following chapters will bear witness to the productivity of this process.

References

1 Crabtree BF, Miller WL (eds) (1999) *Doing Qualitative Research.* Sage Publications, Thousand Oaks, CA.

2 Balint M (1957) *The Doctor, His Patient and the Illness.* Pitman, London. 2e, 1964; Millennium edition, 2000. Churchill Livingstone, Edinburgh.

3 Addison RB (1999) An antidote to physician burn-out: the Balint group as a hermeneutic clearing for the possibility of finding meaning in medicine. In: J Salinsky (ed) *Proceedings of the 11th International Balint Congress.* Limited Edition Press, Southport.

4 Main T (1978) Some medical defences against involvement with patients. *J Balint Soc.* **7**: 3–11.

5 Otten H (1998) Balint-work in Germany. *J Balint Soc.* **26**: 16–19.

6 Courtenay M, Sackin P (1999) Doctors' defences – work in progress. In: J Salinsky (ed) *Proceedings of the 11th International Balint Congress.* Limited Edition Press, Southport.

5

The group works on the cases: threats to the doctor

Michael Courtenay

As we have described in the previous chapter, agreement on the questions used to help us to understand defensive behaviour by doctors did not come easily. They were hammered out and repeatedly modified over many months of work before they assumed their final form. During this period it became clear that considerations of the available time and energy of individual doctors played an important part in what happened during consultations. The following four cases illustrate how the gradual clarification of some of the difficulties encountered led to a better understanding of why the doctors had been upset. We also consider a number of issues such as:

- the doctors' perception of how much time and energy are available at any given juncture;

- how important it is for doctors that patients should respond positively to their ministrations;

- how personal experiences in the doctor's life can determine professional actions.

The cases are analysed in some detail, as this seems necessary for an understanding of the doctors' defence mechanisms and how the group tried to clarify them. Such a discussion would be of limited value if it only applied to the cases under consideration. We hope that readers will be able to apply some of our ideas when they think about their way of working with patients. We don't think that defences are unique to the doctors taking part in the research group!

Diagnostic confusion

Our patients look to us primarily to find out what ails them. Although they look to us for other things, without a diagnosis being made their anxiety remains. Perhaps giving the illness a name represents the last vestiges of the shaman's cloak with which some patients may still wish to clothe us. However, a name implies that we *understand* the patient's condition, whether we do or not. It is only after they have gained some understanding of their condition that patients ask for therapy. The whole process adds up to an implicit contract. The patient expects the doctor to make sense of his complaint, while the doctor expects the patient to behave in a way which seems proper to the doctor in the circumstances. In the background are emotional elements from both patient and doctor.

The word diagnosis often bears a cachet of precision but in practice we use it as a preliminary working hypothesis which can then be tested, to destruction if necessary. The passage of time taken to make a diagnosis is only one of the ways that time enters the equation. Pressure of time in busy practice can so disturb the doctor's equilibrium that the exercise of professional expertise may be blighted. For example, here is a case where diagnostic confusion appears related to the patient's apparent lack of appreciation of the value of time spent with a professional:

I am very ambivalent about presenting this patient. He is a man in his late 30s and an infrequent attender but the consultations are always incredibly time-consuming and seem to lead nowhere. He commutes to the city where he works in a library but he has told me that he can always arrange free time to do other things. He had some peculiar symptoms, as always. But there was another factor leading to this presentation.

About a fortnight ago I had thought I would like to present his case, so I reviewed the notes, after which I thought I had all the facts at my fingertips. But the case went completely out of my mind until last evening, when I was driving close to the surgery. Instead of collecting the notes I rationalised that in a Balint group one is supposed to tell the story out of one's memory store. As it was getting late I drove past the turning to the surgery thinking that I wanted to get home early to get a good night before the group meeting early the next day. I did not want to spend more time on preparation.

Before Ian became my patient he had had an illness about 5 years ago with neurological symptoms, including facial pain and numbness, so he was referred to a neurologist at a teaching hospital. The team there subscribe to the belief that myalgic encephalomyelitis (ME) is a post-viral condition and they gave his illness that label. He seems to have accepted the diagnosis for quite some years. He has only attended our practice five times in the last 5 years, but three of these have been in the last few weeks.

He saw another doctor in the practice on one occasion and asked to be referred back to the neurologist, whose letter dealt chiefly with facial pain. He came back to see me to talk about that, accompanied by his wife who did a lot of the talking, and at the end I felt overwhelmed by his collection of endless symptoms. I had sat virtually silent for 20 minutes without being able to make any connection between the symptoms and the patient's life. His wife was pushing for something to be done though it was not at all clear in which other direction to send him, though an ear, nose and throat surgeon was one of the possibles because he talked of 'sinusitis'. I decided that the only way to stop the consultation continuing all day was to take some therapeutic action. The neurologist had actually suggested that a tricylic antidepressant might help the facial pain, so I managed to get him to accept trying a small dose. He returned for a follow-up and agreed that the antidepressant did seem to have afforded some relief, but he would still like to see a surgeon if the symptom persisted. This consultation only took 20 minutes rather than the 40 of the previous one, but at the next follow-up things were back to where they started. He did not want to see a surgeon after all. There was yet another clutch of symptoms, all described in the most minute detail, presented in such a way that I really had no idea what he did want.

He protested that he was not one of those crazy people who thinks that there is some magic bullet to cure the condition. Nor did he wish to be labelled as an ME sufferer.

This made my heart sink. I felt that he cannot be dismissed because he is being so very reasonable. Nevertheless, he was consuming a lot of my time without achieving any result. But at this juncture he declared that he didn't think he would be able to continue working much longer because he was not feeling well enough to do so. I feel ashamed that I didn't pursue this further but I just didn't understand how his symptoms would prevent him working. Although he said the pain was bad sometimes, he didn't want to take painkillers, and he seemed to be saying that there was some other symptom of his condition, actual or potential, which was concerning him. In the end he agreed to go to see a surgeon privately for a second opinion, my feeling being that it was not right that the NHS should have such a time-consuming patient. He didn't mind where he saw the consultant, saying that he had 'all the time in the world in my job'.

The group struggled to understand what happened to the doctor in the course of these exchanges. It was certain that even if the patient had all the time in the world the doctor did not. It seemed that there were moments in the consultations when the doctor knew, or hoped he knew, that essentially there was no somatic basis for Ian's complaints. However, it seemed that it had not been possible to widen the scope of the conversations into areas which were not rooted in the body. There was a feeling in the group that patients with a very marked somatically orientated view of pathology were unlikely to be receptive to psychological explanations. At this juncture it was pointed out that this view was essentially a generalisation which should alert the group to the likelihood of defensive behaviour!

Although the patient might have thought that it was essential to describe his symptoms accurately to help the doctor elucidate a complex case, his verbosity in detailing his complaints seemed to be foreclosing the possibility of any movement. The group ruminated about how interesting the underlying story might be, while at the same time noting that the doctor's curiosity had been deadened by the way in which the patient had chosen to present it. His wife seemed to be speaking on his behalf rather than her own, though the group had divided opinions about that, some suggesting she felt shut out by him in the same way the doctor did. The fact that, on paper, his CV suggested he would be an interesting person to meet was at variance with his appearance as a boring man to the doctor. This had to be explained.

The patient talks and the doctor listens, but the process seems unproductive. It is as if an apparently meaningful story produces a meaningless pattern to the doctor's mind. The patient talks in what is virtually a foreign language and the doctor seems unable to persuade him to speak in a language he can understand. And the doctor's difficulty was plain even to the reception staff as they included Ian's name on a list of 'heartsink' patients which they served up to the doctor as a joke on April Fools' Day!

It was suggested that the patient might be obtaining benefit from these consultations which the doctor felt were so dysfunctional. The doctor's great capacity to sit and listen, allowing the patient to unburden himself of his symptoms might, indeed, relieve his distress in some way which was not apparent to the doctor. It might even be connected with his thought that he was becoming too ill to work in what, on his own testimony, was a very undemanding job. Alternatively he might fear a more serious cause for his illness. He was certainly preoccupied with his symptoms, and it had to be acknowledged that they were genuinely experienced, irrespective of causation. It seemed that the doctor's calm acceptance of the symptoms might go a long way in communicating to the patient that they were not life-threatening. However, it became clear the doctor often felt that the patient was trying to make him suffer. It seemed that the doctor had as much difficulty in telling the group the nature of *his* distress as the patient did in telling the doctor about his.

How are we to understand this doctor–patient relationship? What is clear from the presentation is that the doctor felt that the patient was in control. The doctor became 'de-skilled' by the feeling that the patient was consuming an inordinate amount of his time. This not only left the professional field in a chaotic state but resulted in the doctor feeling personally bruised and driven into a corner. The suggestion that the patient might pay for a private consultation with the surgeon might well have been dictated by the fact that the doctor half realised that the patient sucked professional time into a black hole.

Diagnostic confusion, then, may be a signal that the patient has, consciously or unconsciously, rendered the doctor's professional skills ineffective by exercising control in a way which is not immediately apparent. An overview of the unfolding story seems to demonstrate that the time factor flows throughout. This is apparent not only in the consultations themselves but even in the preliminary steps the doctor took after deciding to present the case. There seems to be an only partly acknowledged sense that a doctor has only so much time and energy to allot to each patient. If this semi-conscious 'rationing' is challenged, then the professional skills of the doctor may become compromised. Although the doctor was aware of the length of the consultations, it proved impossible for him to 'take control' because this would seem to have run counter to the laudable attempt to be a good listener. This would seem to explain why the doctor appeared to be in such a state of inner conflict to the extent that he felt 'knotted inside' (*see* Chapter 11). Here, perhaps, is an example of an occasion when a conscious defence mechanism is justifiable and the doctor's pain transmuted into a therapeutic interpretation for the patient such as: 'You may have all the time you need, but most of us don't'. While the group felt that most doctors would have been upset by this patient, this doctor seemed to be rendered particularly disabled by him, his passivity being an understandable but ineffective defence against engagement.

Threats to the personal self

Every so often a patient's presentation seems to challenge the doctor's equilibrium, not because of any intellectual challenge in terms of making a diagnosis, but because of a dimly perceived notion that the patient will drain the doctor emotionally if he is given time to unburden himself. Recent advances in neuroscience seem to indicate that the separation of thinking and feeling in the human brain is not possible. Inevitably each of us, as we enter a consultation, brings both rational and emotional elements into the relationship. Perhaps it is not surprising that we may seek to protect ourselves from too much emotional involvement.

Consider the case of a woman in her late 20s who brought her baby as an emergency at the beginning of a Monday morning surgery. She was the wife of a man whose family had been patients of the practice for a long time. Her sister-in-law had on one occasion warned the doctor that she thought the patient was drinking too much:

'My baby's been crying all night, he won't settle, he doesn't eat and he's very constipated and losing weight, here, look at him.' Tina is a striking, tall, blonde girl with a disarming, wide-open smile. I was immediately on my guard. I knew that more than one of my partners had felt defeated in trying to tackle her numerous problems which had included the suspicion that she had an eating disorder. I had seen her once myself at an antenatal clinic during her recent pregnancy, and thought she was laughing and joking in what seemed to be an inappropriate way. I wondered then if she was hiding depression. This seemed to be confirmed when I saw her at the postnatal clinic where she seemed overtly depressed. Later, her sister-in-law reported that Tina was having difficulty in her mothering role, not feeding or changing the baby regularly, letting him cry for long periods and seemingly generally disorganised at home. I realised that the practice needed to get to grips with her problems but had not been her usual doctor up to now.

I examined the baby carefully and found a somewhat underweight baby with an unsmiling expression but nothing else significantly wrong. I found it unexpectedly easy to reassure the mother. She smiled in a disarming sort of way and then said: 'But really you know it's myself, I get very low, weak and tired, and I'm feeling depressed and I feel I need something'.

I felt exasperated. It was only 15 minutes into the start of the working week. Although I ought to have been feeling full of energy, I knew I was getting 'hot under the collar' and could not face that this was the moment to grasp the nettle of her problems. I said to her, 'I've already spent 10 minutes examining the baby and I'm sorry but your complaint is not appropriate now as an emergency. I'd be very grateful if you would make an appointment to come back tomorrow and we'll try and deal with all this then'. I then saw that her eyes were brimming with tears and she appeared hurt and disappointed.

I felt a complete heel but was simply unable to tolerate the pressure of her presence at that moment. It was if I needed fresh air to survive. I had the feeling that I had been mugged but did not know why. She went amazingly quietly but did not make an appointment for the following day. I felt guilty about the way I had treated her but felt I could not have given her any more time.

Pausing to reflect on the state of the doctor's mind at this juncture, it is clear that some of the process was conscious and some was consequent on an emotional state triggering autonomic nervous activity. There appears to have been a conflict between a desire to do the best for the patient and the time constraint on the doctor who, having made time to see the baby as an emergency, was asked to allot yet more time for the mother. The guilty feelings may well have arisen because, during the examination of the baby, the doctor had become aware that the real patient was the mother, while his feelings of 'being mugged' may well have arisen because Tina had used the baby's (largely) spurious ill health as a means to gain access to the doctor at short notice. Although the mother had been bad-mouthed by her sister-in-law, the doctor's health visitor had not confirmed the reports of defective mothering. This had made it impossible for the doctor to dismiss the patient's need for help.

I felt so bad about my treatment of her during the consultation that I was determined to make amends when she did eventually come back. I resolved to try and swallow my exasperation in order to make a fresh start. In the event she did not return until 6 weeks later. She had made an appointment to see me on a Monday morning! She came in with the baby and I felt impelled to pour out a statement of contrition. I confessed to having felt guilty that I had been unable to listen to her problem at that time. Her reaction in terms of body language was one of obvious relaxation. She expressed gratitude for what I had said and then proceeded to tell her story. She recounted how she and her partner had been planning to go away for a weekend and leave the baby with her parents but they were both smokers and she was afraid he would suffer from the effects of passive smoking. Her parents, however, were unwilling to promise that they would abstain for the sake of the baby and a blazing row developed which culminated in them saying, 'Don't bring the baby round'. Tina had sought to heal the rift by writing to them but they had not even replied. She had not spoken to them since that day. Since then she had felt awful and everything seemed to be going wrong. Her confidence in looking after the baby had evaporated. She recounted that things had always been very difficult at home. Her father had bullied her mother, herself and her two sisters to the extent that she now looked on him as a child abuser. She went on to say that she had come to hate herself and could not bear to look at her own reflection in the mirror. She had become frightened that she would put on too much weight and had become fearful of eating. She had to have an alcoholic drink to give herself the courage to go out shopping and was now more anxious than ever because she had to do this more often. I spent a full half-hour allowing her to unburden herself but in the end felt that an antidepressant was appropriate because of the depth of her depression. Interestingly, when I prescribed it, she made the remark that her sister had been prescribed that one with success. I tried to get her to make an evening appointment a week later but she said that it was difficult for her to leave the baby with anyone and so a further morning appointment was arranged.

The next day there was a baby clinic scheduled at the surgery. While I was doing some paperwork in my consulting room with the door open, I saw Tina walk past. Seeing that I was alone she said, smiling, 'I am so grateful to you yesterday for listening to me'. She then took out a parcel wrapped in silver foil and presented it to me. It was a rich fruit cake. 'I baked this specially for you'. I was dumbfounded, all the more so as it was my favourite kind of cake!

Tina cancelled the appointment arranged for the following week and did not request a repeat prescription for the antidepressant.

The doctor was ambivalent about this turn of events. On the one hand there was a feeling that he had met her need (she had said that the she found it warm and comforting that the doctor responded to whatever she said, in contrast to the long silences she had experienced when she had been sent to the practice counsellor before her pregnancy). On the other hand she seemed to have reverted to her untidy pattern of consulting as in the past.

Perhaps the most remarkable thing about the first encounter with Tina was that the doctor felt so bad about what was, on the face of it, a very conscientious approach. His partly conscious defence – deferring the mother until the next day – seemed to make the doctor almost more distressed than if he had got on and dealt with the mother's problems immediately. With regard to the second consultation, the group thought that the doctor's hesitation in getting to grips with the patient's problems was because he was labouring to overcome his defence. The doctor managed to overcome it and to achieve such a successful outcome in one session that the group had difficulty in believing it. However, the evidence of subsequent contacts appeared to confirm it.

There were no further face-to-face meetings and the patient did not see any other partner in the practice. However, the doctor often sees Tina in the street as she takes her son to the nursery. On one occasion he went out of his way to greet her. The group wondered whether this didn't show that the doctor feared rejection by the patient. He accepted this and also admitted that he had been disappointed that she didn't return after the second consultation. He sensed that there was unfinished business.

Challenge to the 'apostolic function'

There appears in many doctors to be a shadowy area where our personal feelings seem to impinge on the rational pursuit of our skill. As a result we behave as if we have revealed knowledge of what is right and what is wrong for patients. It is as if we have a duty to convert to our faith all the ignorant and unbelieving among our patients. Michael Balint called this the 'apostolic function'. It seems to be a combination of accepted traditional medical attitudes and the doctor's agenda in dealing with patients. The former may be entirely sensible but ignoring the patient's agenda is often a recipe for a dysfunctional doctor–patient relationship. This is illustrated by the next case:

The patient is a woman of about 50, whom I have known for years. She is a well-built, pleasant woman with a sense of humour. She is a scientist who has received international recognition for her work. This afforded a special interest in her for me, and I even put 'awarded a medal' on her notes. I've always had a very easy and straightforward relationship with her, though most of the consultations have only been for cervical smears and diaphragm checks. But it did occur to me recently that I knew nothing about her sexual partner.

About two years ago she told me that her sister had had a fatal heart attack. I checked her blood pressure and serum cholesterol and found the latter was raised. I gave her appropriate advice about diet but did not see her again until about 18 months ago when I rechecked the level and found it significantly raised. So I said to her, 'with your family history we have got to treat this seriously'. She bridled at that, which was the first time I had encountered resistance in our relationship.

She railed against not being able to eat certain things she was fond of. She explained that, now her work was desk-bound, she couldn't take a lot of exercise. However, she did promise to follow an appropriate diet. This did not lower her cholesterol significantly so I suggested that she go to the Lipid Clinic. She resisted this for some time but eventually agreed to go. They did the usual investigations and prescribed a statin. She was given a small dose and she was happy with that but when they increased it she complained of terrible side effects so she stopped it altogether. When I was on holiday she saw my partner as she was gaining weight rapidly. Thyroid tests revealed a normal thyroxine but a raised TSH (thyroid-stimulating hormone), so my partner gave her thyroxine, starting with a small dose. However, when urged to increase the dose, the problems recurred. My partner said: 'Your wretched patient was ever so difficult, she won't take her cholestyramine or her statin and now she won't take thyroxine'. I was cross and spoke up in defence of my patient. 'I've never found any problem with her'. I felt rather smug, thinking how I have always said how important the doctor–patient relationship is!

I tried to coax her back on to the straight and narrow and listened to her endless excuses about why she couldn't eat this, that and the other. I asked her to stay on the low dose of the statin (which hadn't upset her) until she returned to the clinic. I urged her to try and increase the thyroxine as her weight was still increasing. She then consulted a herbalist and told him about her serum cholesterol. It seemed that she was willing to take anything the herbalist prescribed, though this resulted in her adhering to a macrobiotic diet rather than keeping clear of inappropriate foods. With regard to the thyroxine, she tolerated 75 μg but when I tried to push it up to 100 μg she came back complaining of 'terrible side effects'. I persuaded her to try 100 μg again when she came back from a holiday but she said, 'I couldn't possibly tolerate 100 μg, I get these terrible symptoms'. I felt my hackles rising. I said: 'I thought we agreed that if you couldn't tolerate the dose you were going to ring me up'. She replied that as it was the weekend I wouldn't want to be disturbed. 'Anyway you'd said that the tingling in the fingers was a side effect of the thyroxine'. I thought, 'I couldn't have said that', but she was adamant.

By now, I was really fed up and I told her so. I said 'How do you expect me to treat you? I'm doing my best, I make the diagnosis, I recommend the treatment, you keep coming to see me to tell me you don't want the treatment. I've tolerated your diets, I've tolerated all these new side effects, I've referred you, I've done everything I can, you know, what do you expect me to do?' (I thought, 'Oh dear, I'm venting all my frustrations on her and I feel very bad about it because I can see she is quite upset'.) Then I said, 'I'm sorry, but I'm sure you can understand my frustration. I find it very difficult to believe that all these effects are due to your drugs, but rather that if you get any symptom you immediately blame whichever is the latest drug that you're on'. She agreed that this could be the case. 'But', she said 'I've got throbbing in the feet since I increased the dose of thyroxine'. In the end I wrote to the consultant telling him that she couldn't tolerate the increased dose. I did it then and there and showed it to her so that she would know I wasn't maligning her. So we arranged a follow-up appointment and parted on reasonably good terms though I still felt bad about what I had done. Later, I remembered that her TSH had doubled its original level which confirmed the need to get her condition under control!

The group discussion sought to understand what had changed between doctor and patient. When the doctor's partner had expressed irritation with the patient the doctor had thought that her partner must have mishandled her. After the recent exchanges the patient had changed from being an admired friend to an annoying pest. Perhaps it was that the patient did not wish to take on a passive, accepting role with anyone. Indeed, the doctor thought that her frustration stemmed from a feeling of loss of control, both in terms of the doctor–patient relationship and also the amount of time spent, but she did not see the way forward. What had made the doctor so upset? The patient had one of the very few medical conditions for which there is a specific remedy. And the remedy itself in this case was a substance that is normally occurring in the body, the very thyroxine which the patient seemed to consider more of a poison than a cure! It was as if the doctor had based the mutual relationship on the basis of the patient's sugar-coated exterior and had not realised what a tough nut lay beneath the surface. The shock and disappointment felt by the doctor were such as completely to destroy her equilibrium.

What was clear about the patient was that, in spite of her apparently worldly success, she felt unfulfilled and time was flying by. She had certainly been bereaved. Perhaps she was depressed. The group suggested that it might help if the doctor resumed her patient attitude towards anything that was brought to her. This had been their relationship before the recent problems. The doctor mused about the relationship. 'I always thought of her as a pleasant, easy, straightforward patient who is quite nice to see but, as it is, I've never allowed her to tell me anything, except about her job and her aspiration to be an artist'. It was a cocktail party relationship. Even birth control checks had never produced anything about her sex life. In fact the doctor was uncertain as to whether she really had one, the diaphragm notwithstanding!

It seemed that the doctor's defence over quite a long period had been to collude with the patient in order to avoid getting close to her pain. Because of her mounting frustration, the doctor became angry and this signalled an end to the collusion, allowing a fresh start to be made. This was confirmed at a follow-up presentation. The doctor now seemed able to contain her evangelical therapeutic zeal, while the patient seemed to have genuinely tried to be more compliant though she had not been able to reach the dosage levels aimed for by the doctor.

The atmosphere reflected a relationship between two human beings who had been able to establish a *modus vivendi* in a professional setting, from which each was able to experience satisfaction, if not perfection. In retrospect, the emotional explosion had revealed the deficiencies in the original relationship and had enabled the doctor to realise that her entirely worthy intentions to make the patient better had foundered on the basis of an unequal relationship. The patient's autonomy had been threatened and had been defended tooth and nail. Backing off not only enabled the emergence of a more mature relationship but actually achieved a more efficient therapeutic regime. Tribute must be paid to the fact that the crisis had not destroyed the essential doctor–patient relationship, showing that even that relationship had its strengths. Indeed, the doctor might not have bothered so much about the issue if the patient had not been esteemed as much as she was.

Sylvia: three missing days

From time to time what appears to be a model of professional conduct of a case suddenly throws up something which appears to conjure up events in the doctor's personal past that seem to play a significant part in the doctor–patient relationship.

One Friday evening after surgery I received a message asking me to telephone the daughter of a middle-aged woman called Sylvia, whom I knew very well. Sylvia's notes had been put ready for me with a new hospital discharge summary pinned to the folder. It read: '?Stroke. CT scan negative. Please refer to psychiatrist'. I reluctantly took the record back to my room and rang Sylvia's number.

Her daughter answered the phone, sounding bright and intelligent. She told me that she had found her mother unconscious in bed and had then called an ambulance. It was uncertain how long she had been comatose and when she gradually came round she had no memory of what had happened. The doctors had thought she had possibly had a stroke but as she had no paralysis they couldn't rule out another diagnosis. They had discharged her as soon as possible. Her daughter then asked me when I could come and see her at home. I was thinking, 'I don't want to go now, it's late and I'm not at my best', so I said: 'Well, how about tomorrow?' 'That will be marvellous, doctor', the daughter responded. So I arranged to visit after Saturday morning surgery. The family have been my patients for nearly two decades. During this time they have suffered many losses. Sylvia's sister died of a heart attack in her 40s, her mother died shortly afterwards and her father became progressively more disabled with chest disease. Sylvia's first husband had deserted her, leaving her with her baby daughter. At about the time of her father's death from chronic bronchitis she met an old flame and they got married. After three happy years he developed lung cancer when he was only in his mid-50s and suffered an unpleasant and prolonged terminal illness. Sylvia had felt suicidal at times during this period and I had to work hard to help her through her grief.

On the Saturday morning visit, it was with a sense of foreboding that I climbed the stairs to the front door. I found a lot of visitors in the well-kept flat, friends and relatives who were gently shuffled out by the daughter so that there were, in the end, just the three of us. The daughter sat to my side, but rather far back so that I couldn't see her face. I had the feeling there was tension between them over the recent events leading to Sylvia's admission to hospital, so that I seemed to be placed in the position of a referee in a game at which I had not been present.

The daughter had apparently found her mother unconscious with wounds on her arm and neck and blood on the sheets. Sylvia was vague as to what had happened but reiterated that the wounds were of no importance while the daughter insisted that there was something to worry about. Sylvia denied that she had been drinking or had taken any tablets but had to admit that she couldn't remember any events for the 3 days before she was found. She confided that she used to see a counsellor but had not done so for some time. She then asked me to arrange for her to see a psychiatrist but it was pointed out that this would mean a wait of some months. The daughter became agitated at this point. She asked me if her mother would be all right on her own and if there were any tablets which might help her while she was waiting. Sylvia then brought up how much she missed her husband, saying she would take flowers to his grave every week. The tension between mother and daughter continued. The daughter was anxious about what might become of her mother if she remained at home unsupervised. But her own work commitments prevented her from being able to stay and look after her. In the end I gave Sylvia a certificate to stay off work for 2 weeks and asked her to make an appointment to see me the following week. I also prescribed one of the newer antidepressants as I felt fearful that she might intend to commit suicide.

There was certainly no evidence that she had had a stroke, being fully mobile and not dysphasic. As I got up to go she suddenly brightened, saying, 'Oh doctor, I'm so grateful to you, you always come up trumps'. And then she said, 'Can I kiss you?' There and then in front of her daughter she kissed me on the cheek, to which I responded likewise.

The group were completely bemused by the story of Sylvia's illness. How could she have been unconscious in bed for 3 days without food and water? The doctor seemed to be avoiding confronting the possibility that she had attempted suicide. It was suggested that the doctor had sought to seduce the group by his long introduction to the case, in which he described the good relationships he had had with many members of the family though, at the same time, many had perished. Was his collusion with the patient's denial of a suicidal attempt an attempt to preserve this idealised image of doctor–patient interaction? Had he been rewarded with a kiss for his collusion? How did the daughter really feel? And how much risk was he taking by his strategy of leaving her at home on antidepressants and a promise to see her the following week?

At follow-up the doctor reported:

In the event, she didn't keep the appointment but she had been seen at home by the psychiatrist who seemed as undecided as I was. He had promised to arrange a follow-up at the hospital and had changed the antidepressant. After a while Sylvia came to see me again. The hospital seemed to have lost track of her follow-up appointment so she asked me to try and sort that out. Then she complained that her right arm felt numb though it had not lost power. On parting she again railed against the higher powers that prevented her joining her dead husband but she had disappeared through the door before I could respond.

The doctor went on to say that he had a certain dissatisfaction with the group's response to this case. Then, to everyone's surprise, he recounted that, when he was 2 weeks old, his maternal grandmother had committed suicide while his own mother was confined in the maternity hospital. His mother subsequently developed postnatal depression. He thought that intense feelings about suicide had had a great influence on his recent contacts with Sylvia. It then transpired that the hospital discharge note which had reached him that fateful Friday evening had actually read '?stroke/?suicide attempt'. The group members all felt sure that the doctor's initial account of the discharge note had not included the words 'suicide attempt'.

Who had forgotten these important words? Whose defences had been mobilised? When the doctor had had the opportunity to refer to the verbatim transcript it became clear that he had not reported the '?suicide'. He agreed that when he was presenting the case his sad family history was close to the surface of his mind. It was likely that his experience of suicide in his own family had somehow made it difficult for him to share with the group the intimacy of his relationship with Sylvia. On the other hand the group, shut out of the intimacy, had made the doctor feel that it wasn't listening to him.

During the initial discussion, the doctor was asked what was really troubling him about the case. He was puzzled, and found the question difficult to answer. Although he strongly suspected that Sylvia's 'missing 3 days' were the result of a suicide attempt, he had not asked her directly (or even indirectly) whether she had tried to take her own life. The tension between mother and daughter (which made the doctor feel uncomfortable) seems to have been due to the daughter's anger with her mother for trying to kill herself. The doctor evidently felt that he had to keep out of this argument. Everything connected with suicide had to be understated and marginalised. Once we know about the death of his own grandmother, this behaviour becomes understandable. Perhaps the anger of the daughter reminded him of his own mother in her postnatal depression, grieving angrily over her own mother's desertion. We cannot know and do not need to know what was going on in the doctor's unconscious feelings. What is clear is that his defences moved quickly in to protect him and there was no question of confronting Sylvia about her suicidal actions. Their collusion was sealed by a kiss. But perhaps the kiss also expressed their warm and enduring feeling for each other and strengthened Sylvia's will to continue living.

In retrospect, there were clear signs that a piece of the puzzle had been missing at the outset. After the first presentation a member of the group had verbalised the problem: 'The patient is puzzling enough but it's the doctor's distress that is puzzling to me'. The doctor's courage in recounting his personal experience of suicide produced the key to the puzzle and it is fascinating that he had no memory of the suppression of the vital word on the discharge summary, somewhat mirroring the patient's 'amnesia' about her lost 3 days.

This case shows the way in which some of a doctor's deepest personal feelings can powerfully influence his professional conduct. We may like to pretend that the 'professional self', wearing its physician's white coat, can operate independently of the 'personal self'. The more we studied our case histories, the more we realised that the two selves are indivisible, and the defences which spring up to protect our personal feelings will often impair our performance as professionals.

In some cases the influence of the personal self is obscure, difficult to detect. In the first three examples in this chapter the defences seem to be there simply to protect the professional self from external threats. The ME patient threatened to swallow up all the doctor's time; the hypothyroid scientist refused to accept the doctor's medical authority; and the young mother, Tina, tried to flout the house rules by insisting on a second consultation for herself. Nevertheless, on closer examination, it is possible to see that there might easily be a personal factor at work as well. Would the ME patient's manner really have upset other doctors to the same extent? Did the scientist's doctor discern something in her non-compliant patient which made her behaviour personally offensive? Did Tina's doctor find that the intensity of her distress rang some sort of bell in the depths of his own experience?

We can only speculate because the personal factors, if they existed, remained well below the surface. In the last case, on the other hand, the personal factor emerges clearly. In the next chapter we shall look at personal factors in greater detail.

6

The personal factor

This chapter will describe three of our cases in which evidence emerged of the importance of the doctor's personal experience in creating and shaping defences against emotional engagement with the patient. In the first case the group's shared realisation of the personal factor remained unspoken. In the second, the group had its first open disclosure of some personal history which the presenting doctor discovered during the discussion. In the third case, the doctor was able to deepen his understanding of his defences as a result of later reflection on his own.

The case of the dapper accountant

This is a case I want to talk about because something about it is very interesting to me. It's not so strong but it's frightening and I'm full of apprehension about it. It's about a man I've seen twice. I saw him yesterday and I saw him 2 weeks ago for the first time. He's 42, quite handsome and looks much younger than 42. A little bit overweight, very nice sort of Boss suit from work, very neat with a tie and white shirt, still looking very neat even at the end of the day. I had the impression that he was one those City/rugby-playing types, you know, healthy-looking. He came in and sat down and said 'Hello' and we shook hands (which I don't always do) but that was something in the way he was and the way I was. He started by saying how he'd been feeling short of breath when he was exercising. He had stopped smoking about 4 months ago and now when he tried to do exercises or jogging he felt wheezy or chesty. He had a sensation of being blocked up in the head as well, the head, ears, nose and throat, that sort of thing. Not painful but not able to breathe very well. I think at that point I said: 'Is there anything else?' and he came out with it straight away: 'I just don't feel well and there's no joy in my life recently and for a while'.

Here we have a 42-year-old doctor face-to-face with a patient of the same age and gender with whom he feels a strange kind of rapport. The patient speaks at first in the language of bodily symptoms and then suddenly switches to describing his emotions.

How does the doctor react? In his own words: 'I accepted that and then I think I went back to talking about his symptoms and I listened to his chest (which was a bit wheezy) and we talked about how your lungs get more sensitive after you have stopped smoking'.

They talked about hay fever and the doctor offered him some antihistamine tablets. After that they were able to get back to the patient's personal life for a while. He told the doctor that he had never been married and had no children but was in a relationship with a woman which had lasted 18 months and the question of 'are you getting married or not' was beginning to arise. The doctor asked him to come back in a couple of weeks for a review of his respiratory symptoms and to talk a bit more about his personal life. The remark about 'no joy in my life' seems to have struck home and lodged somewhere in the doctor's psyche. 'It was a very profound description, I thought, of the way he felt. I was feeling rather worried about what I was going to do with him'.

The patient turned up again, 2 weeks later, 'looking much the same but not quite as neat and tidy'. Patient and doctor shook hands again. His chest was feeling better and they started to talk 'about the other things'. The patient said he found it difficult to talk to his friends about the way he was feeling, but he had been feeling quite bad, he was tearful some of the time and wasn't functioning well at work. He works in some sort of financial consultancy. He has two brothers and his parents are both living but he doesn't really tell any of the family or his girlfriend about the lack of joy.

> He was not actually tearful in the consultation but he looked tearful some of the time. I felt very sad for him, because his life does sound in a very precarious position in that he's 42, working in finance and he's never been married. And he suddenly revealed to me that 6 years ago he had been treated in a private clinic for 2 weeks for stress and depression. He had been offered some group therapy but had declined. We talked for about 20 minutes but it was very difficult, getting things out of him. I asked him if wanted to try an antidepressant and he said, yes, that had been in his mind, something like Prozac to see if it would help. He also expressed the idea that psychotherapy would be too expensive for him. So I actually gave him 14 days' supply of Prozac, which I happened to have in my desk drawer. I also asked him frankly and openly, which I hate doing, whether he felt suicidal and he said, no, quite emphatically. So I arranged to see him again in about 10 days, half an hour before surgery, to see whether we could get anywhere talking about getting him into some sort of counselling. Or whether he just wanted to come and talk to me. Which is the question. I feel he's not going to want to go and see anybody else now.

At this point the doctor said something to the group which gave a strong indication of his own awareness of an affinity or kinship with 'the dapper accountant':

> I think he makes me more anxious probably than most people would be because he's about my age and his life seems not to have quite gone the way he expected and he said that as well.

To other doctors this patient might have seemed a straightforward case of a mild to moderate depression to be treated with antidepressant medication and a course of counselling or cognitive therapy. 'Another doctor' might have briefly experienced some of the sadness coming from the patient – then his professional self would take charge, he would arrange the treatment and follow-up, say 'Good morning' and move smoothly on to the next patient. But our doctor finds himself troubled and apprehensive. The reason seems to be that the patient is like another version of himself, 'about my own age'. But what does a successful established GP have in common with an accountant whose personal and professional life are both faltering?

At first, in accordance with traditional Balint procedure, the group leave this aspect of the case alone. They want to know more about the patient, his work problems and his relationship with his girlfriend. There is speculation about their sexual relationship. Then someone says: 'There seems to be something like a mirror in the way you feel about him. You said, "He'll probably choose to be with me" and you thought, "My God! I don't know if I want to be committed to this guy"'. And the doctor replies: 'I think it's being scared of someone who appears so totally self-confident. And yet he may have a big hole inside. I think I am worried that he has really failed in life and maybe that strikes, worries something in me ...'.

The group continues talking about the accountant. Is he having a mid-life crisis? Can you have a mid-life crisis if you haven't 'had a life', never been married or had children? Somebody says he must have a terribly immature emotional life. Now, everybody in the group is aware that the presenting doctor is gay and that he has never been married and has no children. On the other hand he has a happy and successful long-term relationship with a partner, he is a successful professional, enjoys his job and is financially secure. So, really they have nothing in common, but something about the way the other man, also 42, comes in and shakes the doctor's hand is quite disturbing. It is almost as though the patient is saying: 'I am your other self. This is what might have happened to you if you had been less fortunate'. And it seems to the doctor that there is a fine line separating *his* happiness from the patient's despair. None of this is mentioned but it seems to have been in the doctor's mind, if not consciously, then very close to the surface. As the discussion goes on he continues to hint at the kinship between the two men, doctor and patient. The second consultation was on an unusually hot summer day. The temperature was 33 °C and the dapper accountant loosened his tie a little. 'My fear is (says the doctor) that if you walked into the City now you would see all these people looking so self-confident and they are all falling apart. It's very threatening'.

Is the doctor trying to tell us that behind his own self-confident manner he feels in danger of falling apart? We cannot tell and may not ask. This is not a therapy group, but it is a group which feels free to let its imagination take wing. Now we are speculating about the young accountant's life as a lonely 8-year-old at prep school, writing sad letters home. Someone wonders if he envies the doctor's 'success'. Why does the doctor need to present this particular patient? Is it just the emptiness and the dreariness getting him down. The doctor says he has several patients like this but mostly they are older. This one is different and 'I've got to find out what he's had as a life.'

Someone notes that, in his presentation, the doctor was not flat and depressed but quite agitated. There is some discussion about the fact that the doctor detected wheezing in the patient's chest but did not want to scare him by using the word 'asthma'. Was this delicacy or 'pussyfooting' really necessary? Might the patient have thought that some even more serious diagnosis was being withheld from him? Somehow the conversation gets back to the 'lack of joy' theme. One of the group leaders asks if anyone feels that the doctor was being protective about the patient's emotional state as well as the state of his lungs. Someone detects a fear that the patient might have a soft centre (like a liqueur chocolate) underneath his shiny, confident surface and might be in danger of emotional disintegration. There is speculation about whether the patient regards the doctor as a parent or an elder brother and someone says: 'More like a buddy'. The theme of affinity or kinship has surfaced again. The group wonders whether the patient will return for his long appointment or whether he will just break contact, perhaps with a polite little note of thanks. Someone congratulates the doctor on his sensitivity in allowing the patient to go at his own pace.

 Now it was time for the group to discuss the nature of the doctor's defences with the help of the list of questions. It is agreed that the doctor's concentration on physical examination as soon as the patient revealed his 'lack of joy' was a form of defence against the anxiety which this hollow statement evoked in him. The doctor agreed that concentration on the physical symptoms afforded him some protection and gave him time to think. One member thought that the direct handing over of the Prozac tablets was like a personal gift, a symbolic commitment of care, or perhaps a sweet to palliate the unpleasant taste of the psychotherapeutic medicine: 'Opening this up is going to be painful for both of us, so here is my personal Prozac to make you feel a little better'. To the question: 'Would this patient have upset other doctors?' our presenting doctor replied that he felt he was more vulnerable than most people would have been. 'There's something about being of a similar age.' Someone asks what it was that made him feel so uncomfortable. Was it envy of his success? The doctor replies: 'I think it's because he's asking me what should life be like. And I don't know how I'm going to help him on that matter. Maybe he thought that I was, you know, similar age to him, married with two kids'.

Was the doctor being called upon to disclose what his life was really like – to the patient? To the group? There was a flurry of reassuring noises to the effect that life could be joyful in many ways, not necessarily involving a wife and two children. One person in the group wondered if there was a fear that the patient might have been making false assumptions about the doctor's lifestyle. The word 'identification' is used. Someone says, 'You thought: here's a guy in a suit, very successful – but he was a mess inside. And he's looking at you and he thinks, "Here's a chap married with three kids and a Mercedes"'. Laughter dissolves the tension. The group members agree that the doctor had a specific vulnerability to something in the patient's presentation which made him anxious and hence defensive. That is as far as the group can go within the traditional Balint terms of reference.

Three months later, the doctor presents a follow-up. The dapper accountant came for his long appointment and the doctor learned a little more about his background which turned out not to be so upper class after all. His work wasn't going well and his sexual relationship with his girlfriend seemed to have lost its sparkle. In the course of the next 2 months the doctor saw him several more times and with the help of Prozac there was great improvement. The patient reported that his work was now going well and his sex life was much better. He was still uncertain about where the relationship was going and the doctor suggested that he refer himself to Relate, the marriage and relationship counselling agency. The group took rather a dim view of the referral, feeling that the doctor should really have offered himself as a counsellor. They were also rather scathing about the relationship, mainly because the girlfriend lived in another town, suggesting that the relationship was also distant. This was despite the fact that the doctor said that they met every day at work and spent most weekends together. Nevertheless, the group felt that the problem lay in the patient himself rather than in the relationship and they didn't see couple therapy as the way forward.

When the transcript of this follow-up was discussed at a meeting 3 months later, there was further debate about who, if anyone, should be the patient's therapist. There was a feeling that the patient would not welcome further self-exploration. This led to some thoughts about whether the doctor also felt some reluctance to get more deeply involved in view of the anxiety which the patient invoked in him from the beginning. Who was being protected from pain, the doctor or the patient?

This led one group member, after asking permission to be more personal, to say that the doctor seemed to be unwilling to engage more closely with the patient because the patient reminded him of some aspect of himself or of some way that his life might have gone in less happy circumstances. The doctor deflected this by saying that the patient might equally remind him of certain friends whose lives seemed to be 'in limbo'.

There followed a general discussion about how much the group should seek to discover about the personal and person-specific nature of the defences. There was general agreement that the leaders would provide protection against over-intrusion and that, in general, it was enough to 'flag up' a personal factor rather than trying to examine it in great detail. And there the question of 'how far can you go?' was parked for the time being.

Did we go far enough? One can speculate on the ways in which a more 'therapeutic' group might have used its knowledge of the doctor to question him more closely. They might have asked: 'Did this patient make you reflect on your own life and your expectations at the age of 42? Do you feel secure in your present relationship? Do you miss not having children to bring up? Do you feel there is enough joy in *your* life? And, if not, why not?' Such questions might have been felt as intrusive. On the other hand, in a group of old friends there must be a considerable feeling of safety and a concern not to cause gratuitous pain.

Would 'digging deeper' into the doctor's feelings in this way have given him or the rest of us any greater insight into what was happening between doctor and patient? Our main purpose is to be more effective physicians for our patients. So we need to look for outcome measures in terms of patients' welfare. If as a result of the group discussion the doctor achieved enough insight to be more effective that should be sufficient. This means that he was sufficiently aware of the specific vibrations produced in him by this patient; that he was able to deal with these feelings without being professionally disabled; that he was able to make a judgement about how much therapy he should personally offer. One might also hope that he would be helped by these insights to function with greater self-awareness when he encounters other patients who produce similar vibrations.

In the next case the group was able gently to encourage the presenting doctor to reflect on whether there were any factors that were upsetting specifically for her.

An echo of betrayal

Last Wednesday, when I was on my own in the surgery, my receptionist came and said, 'I've got this woman on the phone, she wants to register, she wants to be seen now and she's been assaulted. Do we take her?' We checked to see if she was in the practice area and she was on the border but just inside. I also discovered that she had been recommended by the local HIV consultant. This suggested that she might be HIV-positive. Anyway, I agreed to see her and in walked a 30-year-old woman with a rather depressed, not wanting to communicate, kind of expression. She came and sat down and said, 'I was beaten up by my boyfriend, my ex-boyfriend, last night. The police were called and they have told me to come along and have my injuries recorded'.

It seems that she had known this man for about 6 months and they'd had a sort of passionate relationship which lasted about 3 weeks – and then she wanted to end it. But he kept coming round, trying to persuade her to continue it. He had come round drunk the night before and made the same sort of advances. When she rejected him he lost his cool and beat her up. She said, 'I've got this terrible swelling here, where he punched me in the face and my arm is bruised, here, where he grabbed me'. In fact, there really wasn't very much swelling or any bruising to see but I tried to be sympathetic. We discussed the police statement and then I asked her about her general health and whether she had had any serious illnesses. She said: 'I'm HIV-positive. It must have been the boyfriend before the one who hit me'. Then I asked her if the man who hit her knew she was HIV-positive, because she bled profusely from the nose. And she said, 'No, he didn't'.

And, you know, I have to say, my attitude to her changed instantly. I was really shocked by the information. And she went on to say that she is on combination therapy so she's obviously got a significant viral load and I found it extremely difficult to continue the consultation. I gave her a note to excuse her from taking her exams but I felt really irritated with her. I kept saying to myself, you mustn't be prejudiced, it's none of your business whether she's told her boyfriend or not. I suggested she see a counsellor. I was getting in a bit of a panic by this time and for some reason I decided she was depressed and I made her be depressed. But she said: 'No, I'm not depressed', looking as depressed as anything. I referred her back to her HIV counsellor, thinking perhaps she'll get her to talk to the boyfriend about the HIV. I bullied her into it. And I gave her some anti-depressants – which I never do at a first consultation – and I said, 'Come back and see me next week'. She came back, she hadn't taken the tablets and I forgot to ask about the counsellor. We mainly talked about the report for the police and whether I would have to tell them she was HIV-positive. I'm thinking of getting some advice about that but what really upsets me about this patient is this total change in my attitude when she told me her boyfriend didn't know she had HIV.

When the discussion of this case started one member thought that as long as they used condoms (which they did) there was no particular moral compulsion for the woman to tell a new partner about her HIV. 'You've got to get over this attitude', he said. This seemed rather disconcerting to the presenting doctor. Another comment was that the patient had walked in as a victim and had suddenly come to be seen as a perpetrator as a result of the HIV revelation. When she heard that the boyfriend didn't know about the HIV the doctor 'simply froze'. Someone in the group said: 'It was as if it happened to you – as if she was bleeding over you'. 'I could cope with the HIV', said the doctor, 'it was the not telling – it's the deceit that I dislike'. Another member asked: 'Isn't there something about somebody who is secretive, quite apart from the HIV, which made you go on the defensive?' The doctor agreed that there might be something in this. She had felt very angry, she had 'frozen' and had started to tell the patient that she was depressed. It was as if, the group thought, she had become unable to deal with the patient as a person and had tried to turn her into a diagnostic formulation (depression) which could be given anti-depressant pills. Another metaphor that came up pictured the doctor at the helm of a sailing boat. She had been tacking against the wind, trying to be sympathetic, when a sudden change in perception had taken the wind out of the doctor's sails leaving her drifting silently.

The group discussed whether the non-disclosure of HIV by this particular patient would have upset other doctors. One member asked the doctor whether the experience resonated with anything in her personal life which would make it particularly painful for her. The doctor then said that when the group had been talking about deceitfulness, she had been thinking of the time when her own marriage broke up. Her husband had told her when he left her that he just wanted to be alone but she discovered, as a result of an enquiry about a furniture delivery, that he had already set up an establishment with another woman. The doctor had been deeply hurt by this deception.

The group was slightly stunned by the effectiveness of the questioning process in this case. The discussion diverted for a while on to the safer ground of the awkwardness felt by the doctor in having to disclose the patient's HIV status in the police report. A little later, someone asked the doctor if she thought this new insight into the 'personal factor' would help her to set aside her feeling of disgust for the patient's deceitfulness and enable her to become more sympathetic. But the doctor said emphatically that she did not think she could bring herself to do that – the feeling was still too strong.

Everyone agreed that the discussion of this case had been a significant event in the life history of the group. We had managed to overcome our hesitancy in talking about the possibility of a defensive reaction having deep roots in the doctor's personal history. Although still a little fearful and embarrassed by our breakthrough, at least we would now be able to say: 'Does this ring any personal bells for you?' and, if so, 'Do you want to talk about it?'

A middle-aged couple

One member of the group reported a case in which his efforts to help a middle-aged couple with psychosexual difficulties were distressingly unsuccessful:

I am never very good at these cases. I'm perfectly happy for people to come and tell me about their feelings, but if they come and tell me they can't get an erection, it always seems to go wrong for me.

They were a middle-aged couple from Turkey. The man has been my patient for about a year and we always got on very well although he doesn't speak much English. He's a terribly nice man, about mid-40s, very overweight, but very jovial, always friendly and smiling and grateful for everything I do for him. Not that I've done very much. I've been trying to help him to lose some weight and to control his blood pressure. Then suddenly he came along with this woman whom he introduced as his new wife. She is about 38 and speaks much better English than he does. She tells me that they have a sexual problem – or rather, he has a sexual problem in that he can't sustain his erection. Neither of them has been married before and neither will admit to any sexual experience. And they wanted my help. I immediately found myself floundering, as I usually do, not quite sure where to begin. He was concerned that his genitals might not be normal so I examined them and, of course, everything was normal and he was pleased about that. So then I asked them what problem they were actually having when they tried to have sex. He was getting a partial erection but could not sustain it very long and had been unable to achieve penetration. I found myself unwilling to embark on detailed Masters and Johnson therapy (which anyway I'm not trained to do). So I advised them just to lie together and enjoy some foreplay and to give themselves plenty of time. I suppose I hoped that they would be able to relax a bit more and nature would do the rest. And I asked them to come back to see me and let me know about their progress. They said this was all very well but wasn't there a tablet he could take which would solve the problem? (This was before the arrival of Viagra and so no such tablet was available.)

They came back the following week and things were obviously no better. I mentioned the possibility of injections but he wasn't very keen on that idea. So I suggested referring them to someone at the local psychosexual clinic whom I knew was excellent. They agreed to the referral and I didn't see them again for several weeks. When they came back it was about something quite different – I think they both had flu. When I asked how the sex was going, the wife said: 'Oh we're not bothered about that any more, we have given up on it, we've come to terms with it'. 'What about your appointment at the clinic?' 'Oh, we don't want to go. It's pointless because my husband doesn't speak good English'. 'But your English is very good, couldn't you help translate?' Then she said, and this is the bit which really got to me: 'We came to you for help but you ignored us and it's too late now, so let's forget the whole thing'.

I was absolutely shattered by that. I knew I had been clumsy and ineffectual but I didn't think I had ignored them. It seemed so unfair. I said so and I tried to resurrect things but she just repeated: 'Forget it, just forget it'.

The group seized on this sad story with great interest and all sorts of ideas were raised. Early on in the discussion someone suggested that the wife might have been desperate to have a baby before she was too old and she might have been more interested in babies than in sex. Then there was curiosity about why she had been so unkind and apparently unfair to the doctor who thought he was doing his best. Was it a cultural misunderstanding? Was she a rather aggressive, 'castrating' sort of woman? What sort of person was she? Gradually it emerged that the doctor knew nothing about her except that she was his nice Turkish patient's wife. It was not even clear whether she was registered with the practice. He had not asked her about her background or her hopes and fears and had not offered to examine her. The group wondered if this had made her angry. Those members with experience of psychosexual work said that it was much more difficult to do in the middle of a GP surgery than in a clinic where there was more time and a different atmosphere. While this was kindly intended, to console the doctor in his misery, it did not seem a convincing explanation of the disastrous outcome. Another suggestion was the fact that the couple were no longer young but still at a sort of adolescent stage in their psychosexual development. This could have been confusing: 'After all, with a couple of this age, damn it, you expect them to know what to do!' The group developed a fantasy at one point, that a marriage had been arranged for the woman who had been very hopeful that she might find fulfilment in marriage and motherhood even at this late stage – and her hopes had been dashed by finding herself coupled with a very fat, clumsy husband who was unable to deliver on the bargain. There was even a joke about an inexperienced army officer and his new wife calling for his 'bearer' to insert the uncooperative organ for them. Sexual anxiety (on behalf of the couple and the doctor) found relief in a little outburst of laughter.

There was some sadness in the speculation that the man might have said to his wife: 'Let's go to my nice doctor, he will know what we should do' – and the result had been a bitter disappointment for them both. Some people saw the wife's reaction as a slap in the face for the doctor that served to release her anger with her husband and her situation. There was general agreement that in some way her suffering had been overlooked for reasons which were not very clear.

At this stage in the group's history we had not formulated any questions about the nature of the defences operating in each case. The question – 'Would this have upset other doctors?' – was not applied and there was no follow-up of the case because the doctor did not see either of the couple again for some time.

In order to understand what happened we need to find answers to some more questions. The doctor is normally someone who takes an interest in his patients' backgrounds and, as he said at the beginning, is happy to listen to them talking about their feelings. He had a friendly, easy-going relationship with the man, so why was he apparently so uninterested in meeting his new wife? He told us that he usually finds problems about male impotence difficult and referral to a specialist seems a reasonable option for any GP. What was the real reason for the couple's (or at least the wife's) angry rejection of this avenue of help? Was she too angry with the doctor to accept anything that came from him, or did she genuinely feel that the language problem would render it useless?

Did the doctor feel that he had gained any insight from the group discussion? Thinking about it afterwards he said that he realised that he had indeed paid very little attention to the wife as a person and it had not occurred to him that her chief concern might be to have a child. The fact that the couple were so mature and yet so innocent had also disconcerted him. When reflecting on the case, he found himself thinking that it was as though he had been asked to advise his own parents on their sexual difficulties. His mother had been 'mature' (aged 40) when she gave birth to him and he wondered if he had unconsciously felt that he was being asked to engineer his own conception! While engaged on this private 'free association' he also remembered an episode from childhood in which his parents were sitting opposite one another in stony silence after a quarrel and he had said to them, 'I don't know why you stay together if you don't love each other any more'. His mother had immediately burst into tears and his father looked very shaken. Their quarrel was forgotten in their concern about their child.

Interesting as these reflections are, it is hard to say how far they can be viewed as evidence of an underlying unconscious 'cause' of the doctor's failure to show his usual empathy. However, he did feel that he would now experience a warning signal whenever a couple, especially a mature couple, entered his consulting room with a sexual problem. Whether the psychological mechanism of the defensive reaction has been revealed to him or not, he is at least much more alert to an area of specific danger for him, which might not be a problem for other doctors. There may still be awkwardness and discomfort but it should now be possible to bypass the automatic, unconscious defensive reaction and engage with the patient as a person.

There was a late follow-up to this case. Three and a half years after the initial presentation, the doctor met the Turkish wife again. In the intervening years she and her husband had been seeing his female partner. Sometimes the doctor would pass them in the waiting room and they would both smile at him in a way which made him think they might have forgiven him. He had kept track of them to some extent and knew that the sex problem had somehow been solved. In the end they had been to the psycho-sexual counsellor – for one session. Her letter reported that they had gone away determined to 'have some fun'. Now they were eager to have a baby (as predicted by the group) but she had been unable to conceive. His semen analyses had been sometimes normal, sometimes deficient in one or more factors. They had raised the money for two private IVF attempts but sadly both had failed. They were now going to a traditional Chinese doctor who had said he might be able to help them conceive.

The wife came to see our doctor to get some information about her blood tests to pass on to the Chinese clinic. It was not clear why she had come back to him for this purpose instead of his partner. Perhaps she did not have an appointment available on the day. The patient was smiling and friendly and the consultation went smoothly. The blood tests were found and the difficulties of IVF were discussed. Then the doctor decided he had to take this opportunity of asking again why she had felt ignored and not helped. The answer was revealing but not very consoling. 'I was angry', she said, 'because if you had helped us to begin with I would only have been 39 and not yet 40 when I went for IVF. The hospital will only do IVF treatment through the NHS for women under 40'. (The timing didn't seem accurate to the doctor, but he let it pass.) 'We borrowed money for two attempts but we could not find anyone to lend us money for a third. So we are going to see if the Chinese doctor can help us.' The doctor wished her luck and she said, 'Thank you, it would be good to have some luck for a change'. Then she said: 'For myself I do not mind too much. We are religious people and I know that in this country it would be difficult to bring up a child who would stay in our religion. There are so many influences against it, not like in our country. But my husband really wants to have a child. So for his sake I would try once more'.

Conclusions

In all three of these examples, there was a degree of withdrawal or withholding of empathy on the part of the doctor. In all three there is evidence that the doctor 'saw' something in the patient that made him feel that it would be unwise or unsafe to get too close.

In the first case ('The dapper accountant') the doctor feels quite warmly towards his patient and there is some sort of mutual recognition that they have things in common. But then the doctor becomes alarmed at the thought that someone so like himself and with a confident exterior could 'have a big hole inside' and actually be on the point of collapse. He continues to care for the patient but does not respond to the challenge of 'being a therapist' for his *alter ego*. The group seemed to be urging him to take on this role but the doctor, while remaining sympathetic, knew that he did not want to get any closer to a man who might prove to be deeply unhappy.

In the second example ('An echo of betrayal') there is a much more violent withdrawal from contact with the patient as a person with feelings. As soon as the doctor hears about the patient's 'deception' of her boyfriend her own emotions 'freeze' and she keeps well clear of the patient's feelings. She quickly turns the distressed person into a case of depression for whom depersonalised pills can be prescribed.

In the third case ('A middle-aged couple') the doctor is so uncomfortable in his role of sex counsellor that he fails to notice that his old friend's new wife is also a person with feelings.

Were these difficult patients? To use the group's standard question: 'Would other doctors have been upset?' – the answer is probably no. Other doctors, in whom these patients evoked no personal reactions, would probably not have been affected in the same way. The other group members act as 'controls' and we can see them wondering why the doctor is hesitating, shrinking away or holding back. Other members of our group would probably have encouraged the dapper accountant to talk some more about himself and his 'lack of joy'. Other members (as we heard) would have been undeterred by the second patient's failure to declare her HIV status. And other doctors would have invited the Turkish wife to join in the discussion and they would have discovered that she was keen to have a baby before it was too late.

Family doctors operate fairly close to their patients as a rule, both physically and emotionally. The doctor's personal self is allowed to flow into the professional self and warm it into life. When a consultation has gone wrong, or leaves us feeling troubled, it is often because the personal self has withdrawn and refused to take part, leaving the professional self to go through the motions without any feelings. When we reflect on these consultations we need to ask ourselves: 'Would this have happened to any of my colleagues?' If the answer is: 'Probably not', then, 'What sort of spectre does this person raise from the depths of my inner self?' We may not be able to identify the correspondence with certainty but it is worth knowing that if this sort of patient turns up again the same sort of difficulty may recur, unless we can find ways to prevent it.

7

How the group reflected on the cases: metaphors and models

Marie Campkin

In any group of people working together there often develops a shared language – codewords referring to individuals or experiences that have significance for those in the know. As the research group struggled to find ways of expressing the feelings and processes which underlie our daily work we hit upon a number of metaphors and analogies which furthered our efforts at understanding and also acted as a kind of shorthand in relating past and present discussions.

Some patients acquired identifying nicknames – the Jack Russell lady, the Californian blonde, the *Tatler* couple – and some recurrent processes were seen in terms of metaphors, of which one favourite was 'the doctor as amoeba' (*see* Chapter 3). This first arose in our consideration of the doctor's personal and professional self in the doctor–patient relationship and its implications about defences.

One case in which this metaphor was applied was 'An echo of betrayal' (Chapter 6). The revelation of the patient's deceitful behaviour in not having warned her partner about her HIV status suddenly changed the doctor's perception of her role from victim to perpetrator. This was so disturbing to the doctor that the extended 'pseudopodium' was withdrawn and the 'indigestible particle' violently expelled, to an extent that the doctor had to retreat into virtually autopilot professional behaviour to be able to continue the consultation.

In the subsequent consultation, the doctor's persisting sense of antipathy was so powerful that we compared it to the amoeba's behaviour in adverse conditions in secreting a protective cyst around itself until the situation improves. The doctor's defensive withdrawal into her professional shell became understandable in the light of the personal issue which eventually emerged in the group discussion.

It may be impossible – indeed undesirable – for this doctor to abandon the protective defences which have been recognised or to ignore the strong feelings that engendered them. At least they are now in the conscious domain – 'bespoke' in Main's[1] terminology – enabling the doctor to decide how best to deal with her responsibilities towards this patient, and possibly to be better prepared should a similar incident occur in the future.

Games people play

The idea of taking part in some sort of game with the patient is a familiar one, expounded in detail in Eric Berne's book of this name.[2] In our work it usually indicated that both doctor and patient were on the defensive, attacking to avoid giving way – and that regardless of who scored the final point both would probably emerge as losers. The analogy often reflected the quality and distance of the engagement. Comparisons with games and sports included 'a hurly-burly like all-in wrestling' and 'a conversation like ping-pong', ending with a smash-shot gesture that nearly swept the doctor's desk clean. The following encounter conjured up for us the metaphor of tennis.

A youngish man, not well known to the doctor, was complaining of chronic, severe back pain. He was off sick from work and his current medication was not helping. The doctor's careful examination revealed no abnormal signs. An orthopaedic referral was offered, but the delay involved was not acceptable to the patient. The doctor offered physiotherapy but even a 2-week wait was too much. The doctor then said he would telephone the physiotherapist next morning (*15–love to the patient*).

The patient was abusive on his return next day, demanding to know whether the doctor knew what back pain was like. Truthfully, but perhaps unwisely, the doctor admitted that he did, whereupon the patient said that the doctor would get preferential treatment anyway (*30–love*). The doctor said if the patient felt like that perhaps he should write to the Prime Minister about it (*30–15*) and the patient said it was the doctor who should write (*40–15*).

In desperation the doctor handed over a large prescription for more analgesics and a long certificate, and was kept awake in the night worrying about the incident and some personal associations it had brought up in terms of past family relationships (*game, set and match to patient*).

In a re-match shortly afterwards, the patient returned in a rage because when he had attended for the physiotherapy he found that someone had cancelled the appointment. He accused the doctor of having done this. The doctor asked 'why on earth he would cancel something he had gone to such trouble to arrange' (*'You cannot be serious!'*). He organised further physiotherapy and an orthopaedic appointment and felt anxious about whether the patient might be abusing his analgesics.

These prolonged rallies had left the doctor feeling completely defeated and de-professionalised. He had been unable to apply his normal expertise either to the clinical problem or to the management of a difficult patient. It was not clear why the patient had behaved in such an aggressive, and later paranoid, way, and the effect he had had on the doctor's equilibrium had precluded addressing these aspects within the consultation.

Subsequently the specialist diagnosed a disc problem and the patient managed to discontinue his analgesics, relieving the doctor's worries about addiction. Some time later he paid a surprise visit to the doctor to tell him he was moving away. His friendly mood was in marked contrast to the doctor's apprehension at the prospect of seeing him. The doctor began by apologising again for the previous difficulties. The patient countered with an admission that he seemed to have problems relating to doctors. The group felt this might be as near to an apology as he could manage. The doctor then took the trouble to suggest a good practice in the new area where he could register, and they parted amicably. There was a postscript later, when the patient had moved away and his new doctor rang up to check on his medication and whether he was genuine or after drugs. The doctor resisted any temptation to score off the patient and agreed the former. It appeared that the patient had found himself a new opponent.

A question which arose from this case was whether a consultation which, from the doctor's viewpoint, is severely dysfunctional, is necessarily unhelpful to the patient. It seemed that here the doctor had come down to the patient's level in admitting his vulnerability as a fellow sufferer from backache and perhaps also in their shared helplessness in dealing with the hospital's appointment system. The patient had penetrated the doctor's defences at a personal as well as a professional level, though we were unsure to what extent he was aware of this. The effect on the doctor was a painful sense of failure but in their final encounter the patient seemed to have resolved his animosity, at least to this particular doctor, despite his admitted problems with the profession at large.

Some other consultations were likened to the intellectual but no less confrontational contest across a chessboard. We talked about the kind of stalemate frequently associated with 'heartsink' patients, where the same moves keep being repeated despite the doctor's efforts to unblock the situation. Sometimes at the start the battle lines were formally set out and opening gambits played ('*pawn to king four*'; '*pawn to king four*').

Someone referred to 'being in an unbearable position – the queen pointing at your king – the attack going straight to the painful thing in you'. How can one defend against this? Interpose a pawn or sacrifice another piece? Perhaps our occasionally noted 'retreat into legitimate professional behaviour' could be an example of the former tactic: change the focus, check the blood pressure, listen to the patient's chest. With the stethoscope in your ears they have to stop talking and it gives you time to regroup.

Something of this sort may have happened with the 'dapper accountant' described in Chapter 6. The doctor had invited the patient to look beyond his physical symptoms but the response was in some way disconcerting. The pause for a relevant but unplanned physical examination allowed the doctor to regain his composure. 'Sacrificing a piece' might involve giving in over a lesser demand, a dubious prescription for antibiotics perhaps, in order to hold the line where a more serious principle was at stake.

We looked for a way of expressing a relationship which was more co-operative rather than confrontational – like dancing, with movement forward and back, albeit with the doctor as the leading partner steering the way. Or perhaps it might be like a tutor–student relationship, which in practice could be played out at levels ranging from kindergarten to postgraduate with different patients at different times.

Another suggestion was of the doctor as shopkeeper, with goods on offer which the patient expects to buy. Whereas some patients seem to prefer the supermarket approach – this is what I want, I'll take it straight off the shelf – others may like a more personal corner shop where they can discuss the relative merits of different products. The doctor/shopkeeper may suggest he has something special which might interest them, or the patient/customer may indicate a need for something that is not on show or in the window. There could be a little haggling over the price but the general effect is of mutual concern and satisfaction.

Responses and reflexes

A different concept which had resonance with our work related to the functioning of the human immune and nervous systems. It is perhaps not surprising if the mechanisms that protect us physically have some counterpart in our emotional and psychological defences.

The nervous system has mechanisms which have their psychological equivalents. The spinal reflex, as the most basic protective mechanism, is acknowledged in the familiar expression 'knee-jerk reaction', denoting an immediate and unthinking response, and most of us could admit to the occasional such experience. Perhaps at its crudest, the patient who comes in with an immediate 'I want' – an antibiotic, a letter for the hospital, an X-ray – tends to provoke an automatic negative response within the doctor, though its expression may be controlled and negotiations opened instead.

Then there is the Pavlovian conditioned reflex, where an oft-repeated stimulus can be used to induce a desired reaction. One might speculate that some 'repeat prescription' patients have got us 'conditioned' – or maybe it is the other way round. The more desirable situation would be a modified reaction under cortical control, adapted to the individual circumstances of the case.

Similarly the immune system is described as having a 'primary repertoire' which is a non-specific defence reaction, and a 'secondary repertoire', which is an adaptive, specific and personal response system developed after repeated challenges. The first could be related to our question 'would other doctors have been upset?', where the circumstances elicited a primary defence reaction, the doctor protecting himself in the face of a sudden unexpected assault, verbal, physical or emotional.

The 'adaptive response after repeated challenges' might apply where a long-standing 'heartsink' situation has led to the development of a defensive strategy on the doctor's part. For example, there are patients whose insatiable needs seem to constitute a 'black hole' into which endless resources of time, concern and care appear to vanish without trace, so the doctor may feel obliged to set limits on his involvement. 'Ian' (Chapters 1 and 5) was a bit like this.

In an individual case such a defence may be conscious, 'bespoke' and probably essential to the doctor's professional and personal survival. On the other hand, a similar strategy might be determined by personal and unconscious factors which may be interfering with the doctor's capacity to deal with a whole category of patient problems.

One of the objectives of basic Balint training, further elaborated in our present work, is to help the doctor to become more aware of his 'blind spots' and to question any 'routine' response to certain situations, in case a defence is being evoked. Once understood, the defensive response might be amenable to modification, or its existence could at least be acknowledged. The way is then open to make other arrangements for patients the doctor is unable to deal with.

One defence we entitled 'principled professional rigidity'. Here, the doctor declares that he or she does not prescribe sleeping tablets, appetite suppressants or some other item. This can be one way of declining a request without enquiring into the distress which lies behind it. A brief lecture on the dangers of addiction, or the offer of a diet sheet and an appointment with the dietician may satisfy the doctor's need to have done something, but leaves the patient feeling uncared for and resentful or even despairing. As an occasional tactic under pressure this may be excusable – as a long-term strategy or a habitual reaction it must raise questions.

In the discussion of the case 'I'd like some sleeping tablets' (Chapter 2) the doctor said, 'There should be a notice in the waiting room: "Dr A doesn't prescribe sleepers"'. It was a joke with more than a grain of truth in it.

How far should we go to protect our principles and our prejudices? Or to what extent may (or indeed must) we moderate our prejudices and bend our principles to enable us to give the patient a fair hearing? On the other hand, does the patient always know best what he wants or needs? Or may it be that sometimes his own prejudices and assumptions have to be challenged? This is where the 'supermarket versus corner shop' dilemma arises, and the customer is not necessarily always right. Most doctors feel that they should be helping the patient to disentangle wants from needs in order to address the latter, and that their knowledge entitles them to explain and advise, though not to demand or forbid.

Group defences and parrot jokes

There were times when we felt that the group itself was exhibiting defensive behaviour, perhaps reflecting that of the patient or doctor who was being discussed. Sometimes this was manifest in laughter and jokes which seemed out of keeping with the serious nature of the case but represented some form of displacement from the pain within it. This certainly occurred with the case 'A middle-aged couple' (Chapter 6) in which the Turkish man's wife accused the doctor of having ignored the couple's sexual difficulties. It was notable that in discussing this case the group became extraordinarily aroused by the problem, for once not interrogating the doctor (who at one point commented, 'You're all ignoring me!') but going into wild flights of fancy about the possible cultural and religious implications, whether it was an arranged marriage – but why so late? – whether the couple were refugees from war, whether they wanted some 'magic' like rhino horn, whether the husband had previously had different sexual inclinations, etc.

We were aware that both the group leaders had had psychosexual training but they weren't offering to share their expertise with the group members. Were they ignoring our needs? (One admitted that he had the greatest difficulty in resisting being seduced into treating the case rather than leading the group, but had managed to 'preserve his virginity'!) It seemed that the group itself was being defensive, sharing the doctor's impotence and retreating into fantasy and jokes to avoid the shame and pain both of the patient-couple and of the distressed doctor.

Despite all these diversions the group did eventually reach a few conclusions. They wondered if the wife felt the doctor had ignored her as a person. He didn't even know her name or if she was registered as a patient, and he hadn't offered to examine her as well as the husband. Perhaps this rather late marriage (of virgins?) had been an attempt to start a family, and the wife was disappointed and humiliated that her husband could not even achieve blood on the sheets to prove her virginity, let alone impregnate her. The doctor's problems in communicating with the husband and his self-perceived inadequacy at sexual counselling had precluded his being a potent doctor for this sad couple. The reaction of the group members was to some extent divided along lines of gender – the female doctors identifying with the wife's possible feelings about being disregarded, while the male doctors were more sympathetic to the husband's and the doctor's impotence.

During the lunch break that followed this discussion, someone told a joke:

A sailor was going on his honeymoon and the parrot which had been his long-time companion begged to be allowed to come along. The sailor was dubious but agreed, providing the parrot promised to behave and not to make any comments, on pain of being sent away to a zoo. On the first night, the parrot's cage was turned to face the wall. The couple were having difficulty getting their suitcase open. He said, 'You get on top and I'll push' – but the lock was stuck. Then he said, 'I'll get on top and you push' – still no luck. So she said, 'Let's both get on top and both push' – and the parrot could stand it no longer. 'Zoo or no zoo, this I must see.'

The association of this story with the case is obvious but the reason for quoting it here is to do with the role of the parrot. There are many 'parrot jokes' where the humour seems to arise from the parrot as the clear-eyed onlooker, free to say the unsayable, to repeat the embarrassing remark, to make a cynical observation or to comment innocently on human behaviour. Perhaps this appeals to us because we ourselves have to guard what we say – censor our remarks to avoid offence, protect our dignity and that of the patient and maintain the correct distance, while the parrot can speak out on behalf of our undefended self.

Unlike the parrot we do become uncomfortable at times with our feeling of voyeurism. We are privileged to be allowed to look into the secret places of people's lives, yet must balance the need for legitimate exploration with the temptations of curiosity and the risk of unwarranted interference. The patient's defences may be challenged but ultimately they must be respected until such time as the patient may feel ready to relax them a little.

This dilemma was mirrored in the group's work, as we began to feel better able to expose and challenge our own and each other's defensive actions in the consultation. Previously accepted limits of group behaviour had been to look at the doctor's case presentation in the context of the doctor–patient relationship, concentrating on the professional aspects and avoiding comment on the personal implications. The doctor was left to contemplate these in private and deal with them if necessary. This is itself a defence, conscious and bespoke, in the context of a group of professionals needing to learn a new skill in a safe environment. In a group focused on the study of defensive behaviour these limits were clearly inappropriate. However, just as the doctor should feel a delicacy and caution when approaching the most sensitive areas of the patient's distress, so we felt some discomfort and apprehension in exploring our colleagues' vulnerability, both in regard to admitted failures of technique and skill in the consultation and still more in their recognition and admission of the personal and private factors which might be relevant to these failures.

The group had to resist the temptation to offer comfort and reassurance in place of challenge and enquiry, but had also to limit curiosity and intrusion beyond the point where the doctor was currently needing to stand. As happens with patients, the process of understanding develops its own momentum and further insights emerge with time, which the doctor may feel prepared to pass on to the group.

Members of the group have shown considerable courage in exposing the professional failings and personal vulnerabilities which are normally hidden behind defensive barriers. Our repeated reminder to ourselves was that defences are not bad in themselves. They are necessary and inevitable but they sometimes need to be brought to conscious awareness and then recognised and evaluated.

References

1   Main T (1978) Some medical defences against involvement with patients. *J Balint Soc.* **7**: 3–11.

2   Berne E (1970) *Games People Play: the psychology of human relationships.* Penguin, London.

8

Patterns of avoidance: the variety of defensive behaviours

Michael Courtenay

'Distance' in the doctor–patient relationship appears to be important. A close relationship is often perceived as a 'good' doctor–patient relationship, though this may just reflect the doctor's feeling that he 'likes' the patient. Whether this improves the patient's care is another matter. While it may encourage the doctor to do something special for the patient it may also result in the doctor being so close to him that he cannot see the wood for the trees. The doctor as a professional has a duty to empathise with the patient as far as possible in the first place, but then must stand back and survey the patient in the context of life (not forgetting that the doctor–patient relationship itself is part of that). Only then can a more truthful view of the patient's condition be made apparent. It is a subtle blend of subjectivity and objectivity, of feeling and thought. However, its subtlety does not make it more difficult, as long as the doctor realises what needs to be done. The effort lies in perceiving that the skills we all deploy in relating to our fellows can easily be yoked to our professional knowledge.

In examining the patients presented during the research we

endeavoured to understand the nature of our defensive postures and why they had arisen. The antecedents to the defensive behaviour were often easier to understand than the nature of the behaviour itself, though that is probably to do with the fact that an explanatory sentence is often easier to compose than a succinct definition. Looking at the answers to our self-imposed second question: 'What was it that upset the doctor?', was often easier to answer than the first question: 'What was the nature of the defence?' There were endless attempts to discover a word that was more appropriate than 'upset', but the group failed to find one, while at the same time still being aware that it was unsatisfactory. One reason for this seemed to be that 'not being upset' often concealed the fact that the doctor was too close to the patient, and therefore blind to the fact that the professional action taken appeared to be distorted by the closeness. Remaining empathic for too long sometimes prevented the doctor from finding the best treatment for the patient.

In this chapter we will revisit some of the cases already discussed in detail and look more closely at some of the defences deployed by our doctors. Perhaps we should start by being clear that these defences are not defences in the psychoanalytic sense. They are 'patterns of avoidance' which may well have a basis in the doctor's personal self but not necessarily so. Let us first take the patient with ME described in Chapter 5. The doctor seemed unable to 'take control'. Instead he struggled conscientiously to reach a diagnosis without disturbing the patient's apparent perception that the doctor had unlimited time available for him. Far from producing a useful result, this doctor–patient contract led only to a reduced understanding of the nature of the patient's illness, with the result that a further referral of doubtful appropriateness was made. Indeed, at the end of three long and exhausting consultations a definitive diagnosis remained as elusive as ever. Had the doctor been able to disengage with the patient's subtle method of being over-demanding, had he adopted a less passive stance, it is possible that he would have recognised the dimension of the doctor–patient relationship that was preventing progress in the direction desired by both patient and doctor.

It is important to stress that empathic engagement, far from being a snare to be avoided, is an essential step while working with patients. It is only when truly 'professional' disengagement does not subsequently take place that problems arise. Take the case of Sylvia, discussed in Chapter 5. The possibility of a suicide attempt noted on the hospital discharge slip was 'forgotten' by the doctor on presenting the case to the group and he persisted in 'protecting' Sylvia even from her daughter's anxieties about her remaining on her own at home. It was only when the doctor felt comfortable enough to recount the tragic suicide of his grand-mother close to the time of his own birth that the group came to understand his reluctance to entertain the idea that Sylvia had wanted to kill herself.

Arguably, the protectiveness offered to the 'dapper accountant' (Chapter 6) by his doctor was to some extent useful. By giving his patient a 'personal' supply of Prozac, he indicated personal as well as professional concern with the intention of easing the patient into a more productive professional relationship. Another patient, the young woman with breast cancer (Chapter 3), also elicited a protective response from the doctor. At the first consultation, the group thought that the doctor had felt so protective towards a patient who 'never gave any trouble' that it became impossible to face the possibility of the lump being malignant. It has to be said that the doctor really did think that the lump was, on examination, typical of a benign tumour, and this led to loss of professional confidence with regard to diagnosing breast lumps.

This brings us to the question of a recurring observation in the research – a perceived reluctance to engage with a patient. The first case in which this element of reluctance manifested itself was that of Tina, recounted in Chapter 5. The doctor's presentation was vivid and charged with obvious emotion. While it was compara-tively easy to defer seeing the patient for her problems after dealing with her child's illness at an emergency consultation, the doctor still felt reluctant to engage when she had made an appointment to discuss her own concerns. He stood, figuratively speaking, at the edge of a cold sea and did not want to enter the water. The spectre of the patient as a difficult and unrewarding person remained before his eyes and it was only when, with considerable courage, he took the plunge that he found the water was not as cold as he had supposed and discovered that he was able to help the patient. What is profoundly interesting is that he then projected all his negative feelings on to the group! So much for the fiction that such groups do not have any therapeutic function.

Another case in which reluctance was manifest was that of the Turkish couple described in Chapter 6. The reluctance here was not as much in the professional sphere as in the previous case, but mixed with personal reservations. The couple were perceived as older than the doctor, and so triggered the natural distaste which would be implicit if asked to give advice to one's parents on sexual matters. Here it is important to appreciate that the precise number of birthdays involved is less important than the doctor's feelings in the matter.

Another recurring theme was 'conflict'. Patients became 'difficult' because their wishes differed from what the doctor thought proper for the patient role. Take the case in Chapter 3 of the man who asked for sleeping pills. This amounted, from the doctor's point of view, to asking for treatment before a diagnosis had been reached. This is not solely a doctor's problem. 'First things first' is a commonly held social convention. Essentially, it is a struggle over who is to be in the driving seat, who has the real power. For the patient it probably seemed a perfectly reasonable request. He was consuming too much alcohol anyway and could not sleep, probably partly as a result of the drinking. However, from the doctor's point of view there were other factors. Somehow the very sight of the patient triggered negative feelings from a past encounter. In addition the patient was engaged in counselling others, which implied something of an equal professional footing that was unwelcome to the doctor's feeling of professional identity. There was, therefore, a combination of negative personal and professional feelings that drove the doctor towards an authoritarian stance.

In another case from Chapter 5, the decorated scientist came into conflict with the doctor in a more subtle way. The doctor approached the new problem presented by the patient in the context of a previously warm relationship, based professionally on routine gynaecological checks, combined with a personal interest in the patient's unusual and interesting work. However, the doctor had not bargained for the patient's health beliefs being as unorthodox as her work. When faced with the patient's unwillingness to proceed down the path of conventional treatment, even in the face of evidence that her condition was worsening, the doctor became distraught.

The prospect of a patient with a thoroughly validated organic diagnosis capable of being treated with specific substitution therapy, who wished to travel along unorthodox tracks of extremely doubtful value, was too much for the doctor. What was virtually a row ensued. The establishment of a *modus vivendi* was only reached after the doctor made conscious efforts to withdraw her strong feelings of professional potency and propriety to a safe distance in the doctor–patient relationship. In the event this manoeuvre yielded good results for both doctor and patient.

There is another defence which is more difficult to label. Perhaps 'manipulative' is the nearest description. A patient, not previously discussed, came complaining of symptoms which she suggested might be due to an incipient menopause. The doctor had known the patient a long time and, although she was not a frequent attender, every previous complaint had apparently been psychologically determined. Furthermore, in at least two previous consultations, the patient had resisted such a diagnosis, but nevertheless ended up in a psychiatric ward. The doctor again thought that the symptoms were likely to stem from emotional tension rather than hormonal deficiency but, in the light of previous experience, she sought to head off a confrontation by agreeing to test hormone levels. The tests showed that the patient was not close to the menopause. When the doctor told the patient, she became incandescent with anger, made a gesture which threatened to sweep everything off the doctor's desk and stormed out. At the next meeting of the group the doctor said that when she had read the transcript of the case discussion she had been amazed at the way she had treated the patient. The group responded by suggesting that the doctor had behaved 'dishonestly' by ordering the hormone tests while concurrently believing that the patient's symptoms were psychosomatic. This was arguably a defensive measure which had signally failed.

Subsequently the doctor was able to address the patient's underlying problem.

Another case (*see* Chapter 1) concerned the woman affected by childhood polio who had opted to have a baby, although severely disabled, and without the support of a spouse. There was even high-level discussion that she was suffering from the post-polio syndrome. She had more recently come complaining of joint pains and the doctor had found himself making a referral to yet another specialist at yet another institution. He repented of this in her absence and when she returned told her that he had considered the problem and decided to cancel the referral. She was very upset and he found himself taking her blood pressure as a means of putting distance between himself and the patient's distress. The patient got up without a word, though visibly in tears, and left the consulting room. The group labelled this kind of tactic as 'retreat into technology', which seems a common manoeuvre in the general practice setting.

We have therefore seen different doctors 'avoiding' a helpful relationship with their patients in a whole variety of ways. These include getting too close to the patient, not getting close enough, behaving in a manipulative way and even being less than honest with the patient. Terms such as reluctance, passivity, overprotectiveness and conflict cover many of the situations discussed. Perhaps we can reasonably surmise that these 'avoidance' behaviours are not unique to the doctors taking part in our research but that they affect other doctors as well. The question arises as to whether there is a relationship between such avoidance behaviour and the deeper defences within doctors. The encounters discussed in detail in Chapter 6 suggest that such a relationship can indeed exist.

During the course of the group it was made clear that there was no pressure to be exerted on any doctor who did not wish to expose any such personal factors. However, group members were all willing to examine their patterns of avoidance with patients and to look in some way at how personal issues may have affected these consultations.

This leads to the issue of counter-transference. Balint group leaders have always avoided using psychoanalytic terms in the course of group work and theoretical aspects of psychoanalysis are never discussed. However, the early group leaders were all psychoanalysts and their teaching about the doctor–patient relationship was informed by their belief in the importance of transference and counter-transference. From the beginning, Michael Balint emphasised how important it was for doctors to study their own feelings during the consultation, and especially those aroused by the patient. He did not use the word 'counter-transference' but there can be no doubt that this was the word he would have used with his analyst's hat on.

Freud originally thought that counter-transference had a dangerous propensity to light up unresolved conflicts in the analyst's unconscious mind. He recommended a lengthy personal analysis to eliminate the analyst's own pathology. Later analysts widened the concept of counter-transference and it came to be seen as a valuable instrument of diagnosis as well as of potential danger.

All views on counter-transference that have developed during the past 50 years have embraced the realisation that the analyst's identity includes a feeling person. He or she has a personal identity as well as a professional identity and both are implicated in the work that goes wrong and, indeed, right as well. The 'feeling person' is not just a matter of professional competence but also of personal identity – the conscious and unconscious role he or she is entering into with the patient.

A number of the cases presented in the group appeared to be clear examples of counter-transference being at work, although it seems likely that it underpins all the defensive postures (see Sylvia in Chapter 5 and the Turkish couple in Chapter 6, for instance).

Consider the case in Chapter 3 in which the deaf patient's hearing aid fell to pieces on the doctor's desk. While it is true that the context of the consultation was not auspicious, in that the patient had been removed from another doctor's list of patients, developments within the consultation rapidly escalated to a point where the doctor shouted at the patient, and not only because she was deaf! The doctor offered the observation that after the crisis of the storm he had immediately felt remorse and, in addition, realised that he was behaving in a manner that was reminiscent of his relations with his mother in her later years, when she too was deaf and somewhat difficult. Having realised that the defences were out of all proportion to the threat which seemed to have been facing him, he was able to see her as someone who needed his help. His attempts to repair the damage (including the hearing aid) were successful in the short term, though the patient selected one of his female partners as her personal doctor. The doctor's professional pride was somewhat hurt, though his relief at not having to cope with her problems offset this, and his insight into the counter-transference dimension of his defence remained as a useful lesson.

Another case also illustrates the phenomenon. The case of the woman who was HIV-positive (Chapter 6) started with the doctor sympathising with the patient on hearing she had been beaten up by her boyfriend. But when the patient recounted that her boyfriend had made her nose bleed but that she had not told him of her HIV status, the doctor was profoundly shocked and her attitude went into reverse. The doctor had genuine difficulty in continuing the consultation because of the intensity of her feeling that the patient had treacherously put the life of her ex-boyfriend at risk, albeit that he had been violent when rejected. When the group suggested there was no overriding moral compulsion to tell a new partner about one's HIV status provided condoms are used, the doctor was disconcerted. After a brief pause she shared with the group her own story of betrayal, when her husband deserted her for another woman. Although this was a case of a woman betraying a man, in the doctor's mind the similarity with her own painful experience came to the forefront of her consciousness.

A third case, not previously discussed, may also illustrate the counter-transference defence. A West Indian woman, a single parent with two daughters, had been badgering the doctor over some years with many complaints. Eventually the patient had a hysterectomy for dysfunctional uterine bleeding. The younger daughter became pregnant at about the same time and it was in dealing with her that the doctor came to realise that the family was highly intelligent, the elder daughter having recently gained a degree. The doctor then understood that he had been stereotyping the family in a rather dismissive way, and came to a conscious resolve that 'he must love the patient (the mother) more'. He reported that his change of attitude towards her revolutionised the warmth of the relationship, the patient eventually saying to the doctor that she 'didn't know how he had tolerated all her comings and goings'. The doctor then told the group that he had come to realise that some of his negative feelings towards the patient may have originated in the fact that his father had divorced his mother to marry a black woman.

Traditionally, Balint groups, at least in the UK, have focused entirely on the relationship between doctor and patient. The discussion may well include ideas about the psychological state of the patient but personal and psychological issues relating to the doctor (operating as one half of the doctor–patient relationship) would be ruled out by the leader. Tom Main's challenge, taken up with enthusiasm by the research group, had led to questioning whether this taboo should be broken. This development was seen as a necessary one in attempting to understand the nature of doctors' defensive behaviours. It was seen not as a threat to the basis of the Balints' work but as a logical development of it.

However, we must recognise that only a minority of doctors will wish to spend time in a Balint group exploring the personal roots of their defensive reactions to patients. Do we really need this kind of self-examination in order to recognise our unwanted defences and modify them appropriately? We will consider this question later. Chapter 9 considers some factors which may predispose doctors to deploy their defences too readily.

9

Predisposing factors

General practitioners probably perceive that time is the most significant external pressure inhibiting their work with patients. There are examples of time pressures in many of the cases already discussed but the topic will be dealt with in detail in the next chapter. In this chapter we consider some other common factors which predispose to overdefensive behaviour.

Practice policies

A member of our group working in a fairly deprived area presented a case:

I'm going to start away from the case. The context feels to be part of it – the huge amount of pressure we're under in the surgery. We have a walk-in morning surgery. Sometimes there are no seats in the waiting room and the place is absolutely heaving. We've been discussing it and the partnership came up with a decision which I'm not at all happy with. Patients are to have a choice of three things. They can come to the walk-in surgery, possibly wait a long time but they will get seen. Alternatively, they can book a normal 10-minute appointment within 48 hours or a 5-minute appointment the same day.

I feel caught up in this situation. It partly arose because one partner sees an awful lot of patients. When I click on the computer and I see the number of patients he sees compared to the number I do, I feel ashamed. It is partly to get a fairer balance within the practice that we've brought in this new system and I accept that but I was sort of upset that the whole of my life I've never had enough time to talk to patients and now I shall have even less. I feel that at the end of my practising years there's going to be more and more pressure. So, on the first day of the new system I was feeling pretty stressed. I had the walk-in surgery first, then 10-minute appointments and then 5-minute ones at the end. It seemed like doing three surgeries instead of one. And this was the first patient of the day.

She was a 14-year-old girl, immature. In her school uniform she looked more like 10. The first thing she said was, 'Will you have to tell my parents I'm here?' I said, 'Well, you are under age so you should be here with your parents' consent but I'd rather you told me what it's about. If you don't want me to tell your parents I won't because it's better that you come and talk to me'. The she said, 'I'm worried that I may be pregnant'.

As you can imagine, that was the beginning of a very long story. I vainly tried to establish when intercourse had taken place and whether post-coital contraception would be appropriate (or was being asked for). Soon, I found myself involved in a nightmare discussion of possible rape, possibly by several boys, possibly on more than one occasion. The girl did not want to tell her parents because 'they had called the police before and I don't want to go through that again'.

I didn't know how much of the story to believe and I already had visions of appearing in court for mishandling the situation. I was worried about the risk of pregnancy, the risk of sexually transmitted disease, the impossibility of seeking forensic confirmation of rape, the dilemma about confidentiality and the fact that a quarter of an hour had already passed.

I decided to give her post-coital contraception but, despite the time, went to talk to one of my female partners, perhaps thinking that a break would clear my head. My partner supported my view of the importance of maintaining the confidential relationship. When I returned I explained about the prescription and offered that either I or my female partner would examine her to see if she had been hurt. She declined. She also at this stage refused a referral for a forensic examination by a hospital specialist.

I said to her, 'You did the right thing in coming. I'm not your parent but I'm acting as if I were, doing what is in your best interests, and you must come back and see me next week'. I made the appointment myself. I felt that I wanted to put my arm round her but I thought I must be careful, this girl will sexualise my behaviour. So, the nearest I could come was by verbalising something about being like her parent.

The main theme of this book is the defence mechanisms that doctors employ in order to cope with the distress of their patients. The previous chapters have examined in detail how certain patients make their doctors anxious and how those doctors cope with this anxiety. Our hope, and belief, is that doctors and other health professionals, can modify their coping mechanisms so as to lead to a better outcome for the patient without causing too much pain for the doctor. Clearly, it is too simplistic just to consider the doctor and patient in isolation. There are numerous other factors which can affect the consultation. In this case time was an important factor but perhaps not the major problem. It was, as the presenting doctor said, 'the whole context'.

The discussion of this case was one of the longest we had. The group, in sympathy with the presenting doctor, began by rebelling against the idea of 'conveyor belt' medicine. But was this really what the doctor was doing? He was clearly sensitive to the needs of his practice population and to the necessity for fairness within the partnership. The turmoil of conflicting priorities within his mind somehow seemed to be reflected in the chaotic story emerging from the patient. Arguably the practice policy was a 'defence' against too much involvement with patients and the doctor was torn between his loyalty to his practice and his own need to engage much more fully with patients. Incidentally, the doctor later felt that there was also a personal element in this case as he kept being reminded of a disturbing recurrent dream, associated with the feeling of a terrible event (suppressed in his memory) that had occurred in his childhood.

During the discussion there was a feeling that, despite the doctor's conflicts, the patient was quite relieved. As one group member, slightly tongue in cheek, remarked, 'She got what she wanted. She said, "I think I might be pregnant". The doctor said, "Fine, here are some pills to stop you getting pregnant anyway"'.

Who knows, perhaps some other doctor *would* have had a 5-minute consultation with this girl, simply dealing with her opening request at face value. Such a 'defended' doctor might arguably be better adapted to the 'real' world of inner-city general practice than the hapless presenting doctor.

The dumping syndrome

Another doctor in our group was also nearing retirement. She described how, in her practice, the duty doctor is responsible for seeing unbooked cases but that other partners will normally help out when they have finished their booked cases. However, on one particular morning our reporting doctor saw over 20 unbooked cases. She felt a bit aggrieved that her partners did not help even though she acknowledged that they needed to be finished by lunchtime when they were due to interview two candidates as potential replacement partners for her! In fact the doctor had even made time during the morning to talk to one of the applicants. What was more disturbing was that the last three consultations had not gone well because of the time pressure. She had finished the surgery not only late but also upset and frustrated.

The doctor continued:

The next day I had finished my morning surgery, having seen several extra patients to make things easier for the duty doctor. I could have gone home but decided to stay and do a bit more paperwork. The most junior receptionist rang and said, 'Would you mind seeing this patient?' I said, 'Isn't my partner supposed to be seeing emergencies today?' 'He's busy.' So I cleared the desk and I went out there to find out. I didn't say I'd see the patient, I just said I'd come out and find out what was happening. I thought the partner on duty was seeing a patient but I discovered later that he was actually chatting to the practice manager.

Suddenly I found myself really angry, not something that I'm used to. Of course it wasn't just because of that morning but the previous one, when I'd been left with all that work. I wondered about telling reception that the patient would have to wait till the duty doctor had finished but I had no idea how long his meeting would go on for and it seemed unfair to take it out on the patient. In any case I knew that if one of the more experienced receptionists had been there, this situation would not have arisen. So I called the patient through. She was about 18 and had a sore throat. She was not ill or febrile and it appeared to be a mild viral infection. I followed my usual custom in trying to explain why this did not require antibiotics. Although the girl was not English she seemed to understand what I was saying but was clearly not happy with it. So she brought in her mother (who didn't speak English) and I repeated my explanation, adding that on the basis of many years' experience I was treating her just as I would treat myself or a member of my family. As far as I'm aware this was all said in a pleasant and friendly manner, though it may not have corresponded with their cultural expectations. Anyway, they remained dissatisfied.

Normally I can recognise when it is time for a tactical retreat. I should have given in gracefully, given her some penicillin and gone home. Perhaps all the more so as my habitual attempts at patient education over many years no longer had any personal relevance. If this patient were now to expect antibiotics for her next ten sore throats it wouldn't be my problem. In the event I seemed to have got boxed in to the extent that I could not extricate myself. I therefore left the room and found my partner (whose meeting had already finished). I just said, 'You'll have to see this patient. I'm sorry, I can't, I'm stuck with her, she wants some antibiotics'. He agreed and no doubt disposed of the problem in 2 minutes by giving her what she wanted.

When I went back to my room I just felt I wanted to cry, which is most unusual for me. Certainly if somebody had come in and said something nice to me I would have cried. It seemed that for 2 days running I'd found myself completely unprofessional and out of control and I just didn't know what to do with it. Not only had I not been able to cope with this 'simple' consultation but there were the problems with yesterday's consultations as well. Fortunately when I got home my daughter was there and I was able to get the whole thing off my chest.

The group pointed out that it would be regarded as very 'normally' defended behaviour for a GP to prescribe penicillin to such a patient when the doctor was keen to end the consultation quickly. In this case the doctor was unable to call on such 'normal' defences. Her inner turmoil, no doubt related to her feelings about her imminent retirement, her relationship with her partners and the stresses of the previous morning's work, prevented this. These internal messages completely drowned out whatever the patient was trying to say. At the same time as being unable to harness a 'normal' defence, the doctor was *too* defended, or just distracted, to hear anything about the patient's point of view, what the sore throat actually meant to her, why she wanted penicillin, what other options she might have considered, etc.

The doctor wondered if her partner thought she was 'losing her marbles – and perhaps so did I'. In fact, she quickly recovered her professionalism and continues to work after 'retirement' as the highly competent and empathic doctor she always has been. Her presentation was undoubtedly an extreme one, but it starkly illustrates just how easily background factors can profoundly affect our work with patients. Ultimately the presenting doctor *was* professional in that she painfully recognised her inability to be an effective doctor to the patient and so got a colleague to see her. In less extreme situations we can help ourselves to become more effective by being in touch with our own background feelings and attempting to put them to one side so that we can concentrate on the patient. These background feelings may have been sparked off by the previous patient. Neighbour[1] suggests that at the end of each consultation the doctor may need to do some 'housekeeping', to engage in some distracting behaviour so as to avoid inappropriate feelings spilling over.

We dubbed the case just discussed an example of the 'dumping syndrome'. How irritated we feel if a patient seems to be 'dumped' on us (just the sort of generalisation which signals defensive behaviour!). The lady with the disintegrated hearing aid mentioned in Chapter 3 is another case in point. Many other situations can predispose to defensive behaviour. An obvious example is the angry patient. Curiously, few such cases were presented in our group, the man who roundly defeated his doctor at 'tennis' (Chapter 7) being one of the few examples. Perhaps such patients are those who would upset most doctors and therefore do not require the use of 'bespoke' defences.

Keeping a distance

After some background information about a pregnant patient (who had been infertile) and her husband, one of the most moving presentations we had in the group continued:

> I was alone in the surgery one Wednesday evening clearing lots of admin. work as I often do on Wednesdays. There were lots of letters. There were two from a consultant obstetrician about this woman. The first said that ultrasound had suggested that her baby was anencephalic and, if this was confirmed, a late termination would be advised. The second, written a week later, baldly said that termination had been carried out at 24 weeks. The consultant said he would see the woman in 2 weeks, before her return to Australia where her husband was currently working. These bald letters gave me the creeps, sitting as I was alone in the surgery at night.

In later reports, group members got the impression that only the doctor had been upset by this terrible story. The patient returned to Australia without contacting the doctor and seemed to 'get over' the episode with little trouble. In fact, much of the communication between this patient and the doctor was by fax. She had initially booked to have her baby in Australia. At one point earlier in the pregnancy she had a hospital admission and wanted to claim on her insurance, so she faxed through a request for a letter from the doctor in England. Over the following years several similar requests came through and there was only very occasional face-to-face contact with the doctor. Yet at some level the patient was clearly 'in need' of the doctor. She could easily have dropped any contact and seen any doctor when she was visiting home.

There were several follow-up reports about this patient and the theme nearly every time was of the doctor's concern for her vulnerability which the patient did not acknowledge. Her overt need for the doctor was invariably for some technical reason and not for any emotional support, a situation which made her sensitive doctor feel most uneasy and, on more than one occasion, caused the doctor to 'forget' to do things for this patient that were quite uncharacteristic. Somehow, the fact that this patient did not fully engage with her doctor was more threatening than if she had been over-demanding or angry. The doctor's unease, in fact, had its origins before the awful episode of the termination. Her first contact with the patient was on a weekend home visit to her husband for 'trivial' chest pain. The doctor was struck with the 'perfection' of this charming young couple, straight out of the *Tatler*. Perhaps this had already triggered the doctor's unconscious defences and made her wary about getting too close. It was almost as if the doctor was mirroring the patient's need to keep a safe distance.

If we sometimes find it necessary or desirable to keep a safe distance from our patients many of us are nevertheless alarmed by the growth of more impersonal ways of seeking medical care. Telephone consultations through NHS Direct, walk-in centres or even e-mail correspondence are beginning to replace traditional consultations. At the same time, GPs are expected more and more to engage in activities such as clinical governance or membership of a primary care group (PCG) which take them away from their patients. This is the ultimate in defensive behaviour! But it leaves most of us feeling uncomfortable. Like the last doctor we feel that patients' 'needs' must often be met in a more personal way even if their 'wants' are for a quick fix. There are difficult conflicts between accessibility and effectiveness, between measuring performance and actually performing, and between the individual and the population. These dilemmas join the personal factors we have discussed in earlier chapters as important background influences on our consultations. The final chapters look at how we might be able to overcome them and give our patients the attention they deserve.

Reference

1   Neighbour R (1987) *The Inner Consultation*. Kluwer, Lancaster.

10

The time problem

But at my back I always hear
Time's wingèd chariot hovering near

Family doctors are haunted by the spectre of time. Unlike the ardent lover in Andrew Marvell's poem,[1] the doctors are not anxious to consummate their relationship with a loved one (except perhaps the one waiting patiently at home). The doctor's chief concern is that the patient he is with at the moment will take up more than his ration of time and the queue of other patients waiting will grow longer and more restless. There is also the ever-present threat that the receptionist will add on some 'extras' to the list. There may be an interruption from the telephone summoning the doctor to an urgent visit. The surgery is bound to end late yet again .... In a number of the cases discussed in this book shortage of time has been a critical factor in preventing the doctor from feeling available to share and experience the patient's feelings. If the story needs a long time in the telling, and the intensity of emotion suggests that it will be interrupted only with difficulty, the doctor becomes anxious. His precarious timetable is threatened. Too many consultations and other tasks have already been crammed in and it will only take one tearful outburst or one lengthy hypochondriacal rumination to throw the whole delicate mechanism out of order. The doctor thinks: 'The patient in front of me looks depressed but if I ask him how he is feeling he might start to tell me and then I would be stuck with him for half an hour. I can't cope with that today ...'.

If a consultation goes towards half an hour the doctor may not hear a wingèd chariot but he is certainly aware of the other patients piling up outside in the waiting room and the receptionist stacking up the phone calls and messages which will face him when, if ever, he emerges. He begins to feel symptoms of panic. His defences click into place and he becomes impervious to the effects of the patient's emotions.

External time pressures in the NHS

Why do we have such an obsession and such a problem with time? It does not seem to bother family doctors in other west European countries or in North America in quite the same way. But we are unusual in having a National Health Service and that is the obvious place to start looking for the reason. Shortage of time was probably built in to the NHS from the beginning, although unwittingly. Ours is the only healthcare system where family doctors see their patients entirely free of charge at the point of contact. Citizens of other prosperous countries can reclaim on their insurance to a greater or lesser extent (assuming in the case of the USA that they can afford insurance) but this is not quite the same. Our patients can come to see us and bring their children without paying us anything directly, and over 80% of the items we prescribe for them are also completely free. Most doctors and patients think this is a good principle which should be preserved. Direct payments at the time of consultation would act as a financial disincentive to seeking healthcare. This would inevitably penalise the less well off and restrict their access to a service of which they may be in serious need.

Our service is not only free at the point of need but it is remarkably inexpensive compared with the money spent on healthcare in insurance-based systems. So one obvious solution to the time problem would be to provide more doctors and hence more appointment time. Unfortunately, politicians of both major parties are convinced that the people of our country would be outraged if asked to pay more in taxation towards their healthcare. So instead they look for solutions which will not cost more or not very much more. These have taken the form of ways of reducing access to face-to-face contact with one's own doctor. The patient seeking help may first be assessed by a trained person who speaks to them on the phone and decides whether they need a doctor, a hospital or merely a few words of advice and reassurance.

Recently, general practice has gone through changes which tended to increase the number of patient attendances. We now invite people to come for immunisation, screening and other health promotion sessions. We have taken over from the hospitals a large part of the work of supervising chronic illnesses like hypertension, diabetes and asthma. On the other hand we have expanded primary care teams with highly skilled members such as practice nurses to help us. Partnerships are larger. The chances of seeing the doctor you might regard as 'your own doctor' seem to get less and less – especially if your doctor is on the PCG board or studying for a mind-refreshing MSc. There is a growing feeling that the doctor should be spared exposure to 'trivial' illnesses. These can dealt with by the nurse who will be trained in 'triage', the skilled separation of those who 'need' to see the doctor from those who do not. The government has schemes such as NHS Direct, which provides triage by telephone, and walk-in centres for those unable or unwilling to wait for an appointment at the surgery. Perhaps these measures will lighten the load, enabling the family doctor to breathe more freely and to concentrate on the patient in front of him without worrying about time. There are certainly gains from this approach but there are also losses, particularly for those who still value the tradition of personal doctoring. When general practice was reinvented in the interests of providing an excellent vocational training in the 1960s one of the key principles was that the doctor should get to know all the families on his list personally. That meant that he would know who was related to whom and have some familiarity with the life stories of those families and their individual members. Patients who came with 'trivial' symptoms such as strange pains or unaccountable feelings of tiredness might, if encouraged, begin to talk about what was really disturbing them. Trainees were taught to make a diagnosis in three dimensions, physical, psychological and social. This contrasts sharply with the partitioning science of triage which places each patient in one of three categories: trivial, serious, desperate.

Does 'triage' help?

So far there is no sign that these changes have actually reduced the time pressure in the surgery. It is true that the length of the time slot allocated to each patient has increased in most practices since the 1960s. At that time 5 minutes per person was quite usual and some had to make do with even less. Some enlightened practices were beginning to insist on 10-minute slots and someone calculated that the average was 6 minutes. Hence, the catchy title of a book published in 1973 by Enid Balint and her colleagues, *Six Minutes for the Patient*.[2] More recently, painstaking research has shown that 10-minute slots result in better clinical outcomes, fewer repeat visits for the same complaint and greater satisfaction for doctors.[3] Ten minutes here means the length of a slot which has to accommodate the face-to-face conversation between doctor and patient, physical examination if required, the filling in of forms (now frequently required) and the writing up of notes, either manual or electronic. The patient may still not get more than 6 minutes of face-to-face attention from his doctor. This may be contrasted with 15–20 minutes in continental Europe and 30 minutes in Scandinavia and Canada. In the USA, ironically, doctors are now beginning to feel time breathing down their necks a little more heavily because managed care schemes are pressing them to see more patients per hour and save money.

Is the standard 10-minute system working? Obviously it is not, because family doctors are still complaining to each other and to the media about the stress they are under from the pressure to see too many patients. Patients are complaining, not because the encounter with the doctor is too short – they are accustomed to that – but because they now have difficulty in getting any appointment within a week. What about the emergencies or those who feel that they are in serious danger? Practices have devised all sorts of ingenious systems to get round this. Some surgeries have slots reserved for emergencies, some sessions are walk-in surgeries where, as in ancient times, there are no appointments and it is first come first served. The doctors take turns to do the 'walk-ins' and they dread them. The numbers are too great and time with the doctor shrinks back to 5 minutes or less. So the relaxed 10-minute appointment (for those who have secured one) has been purchased at a cost.

Now, if you are a patient you might think even 10 minutes is not very long. Is my doctor really seeing so many patients in a day that he can afford each of us no more than that? Why not 15 minutes? Why not 30 when there is a need for more? Clearly it is possible to give some patients longer time, but a wholesale length-ening of appointment times would mean reduced list sizes and a corresponding drop in income which would be unacceptable to most GPs. Indeed, such a drop in list sizes, without an increase in the number of GPs, would eventually result in patients having difficulty getting a doctor, let alone an appointment.

Perhaps we should leave the gloomy economics of the time problem and look instead at what *can* be achieved, and is being achieved, within the present constraints. Do we really need to be so anxious about the slipping away of time that we are unable to connect with our patients' feelings?

Let us recognise that nearly every doctor has at some point spent a very long time with a patient in great distress, perhaps someone who has been bereaved and in the care of whose dying partner the doctor had been deeply involved. The patient has a lot to say and to ask, he is very emotional and it seems important to stay with him for as long as it takes. This is more important than whether the surgery runs to time or even whether the whole struc-ture of the doctor's day is wrecked. Sometimes a patient collapses in the surgery with a serious physical illness or the doctor is called out to an emergency at home – right in the middle of the surgery. Somehow, the sky does not fall in on these occasions. True, some patients get restless. One or two may complain, some are kindly seen by colleagues, some decide to go home and some continue to wait patiently. The doctor is not particularly anxious. He may even be slightly elated with the feeling that a good job has been done. If we return to the distressed patient in the surgery, he was probably someone the doctor knew well or had taken an instant liking to. If the patient is someone the doctor feels comfortable with and whom he really wants to help then it becomes possible to become emotionally engaged and not to worry about the passage of time.

Patients who make doctors look anxiously at the clock

Let us now take another look at some of our cases in which the pressure of time seems to have been responsible for the doctor raising his defences and withdrawing his empathic personal self from contact with the patient.

In the case of the lady with the disintegrating hearing aid (Chapter 3) one of the doctor's most powerful (and irrational) fears was that he was going to be trapped forever by a patient who was oblivious of the time she was consuming. Not only would he have to sit and deal with her endless series of demands, but he could not even begin to deal with them until he had mended her hearing aid. So it seemed in the nightmare world into which the unfortunate doctor was plunged. Or did he plunge himself into it? If he had been a little more aware of his personal difficulties with old ladies he might have paused to reflect on his own emotions. He might have realised earlier in the consultation that help could be enlisted to repair the hearing aid, the old lady's anxiety tolerated and her needs met in a more gradual succession. He did realise all this eventually but not before he had caused a good deal of distress to his patient and himself. The real problem was not the eating up of his precious time but his difficulty in coping with someone whose personality was painfully familiar from his own inner world.

In the case of Tina (Chapter 5) the doctor dealt with her baby (which took 15 minutes) and then it became obvious that Tina herself had a huge burden of distress to unload. It was the first consultation of the day, already the timetable had begun to slide out of control and now the doctor seemed to be faced with an added consultation that threatened to take up two or three more of the precious 10-minute slots. But was it just the pressure of time or was there something about Tina herself and the depth of her distress that struck him like a flash of lightning? Perhaps he instantly recognised something at an unconscious level which he knew would affect him deeply. He says that he felt he 'had been mugged', which suggests a violent assault on the emotions. He rapidly withdrew his personal self from harm's way and told Tina firmly that she would have to come back the next day. We know that this is a doctor who is usually willing to spend a long time with distressed patients. He has been in practice too long to be worried about slipping timetables. He must know that even if your day is ruined you will survive. If this patient had been a different person – perhaps not someone who was crying with a baby in her arms – then the doctor might have let the timetable go hang and listened with attention and sympathy as he normally does. Fortunately, he was eventually able to redeem the situation and was rewarded with a cake. General practice is generous in the opportunities it provides for us to put things right and repair the damage we have done.

In the case of the man with ME (Chapter 5) the first consultation lasted for 40 minutes. The patient droned on and on about his symptoms in a way that made no sense to the doctor. It seemed that his precious time was being relentlessly chewed up and swallowed by the patient with total disregard for the doctor's discomfort. If the content of the patient's discourse had been more interesting or useful it might have been possible to engage with him and have a conversation. Instead, it was like being forced to listen to a tedious and utterly incomprehensible lecture. We are always more painfully aware of the passage of time when we are bored or angry. When the patient is likeable and easy to sit with, when we can share their distress without too much personal pain, the clock ticks more softly and we are less conscious of it. When the patient is difficult or arouses negative feelings for (often obscure) personal reasons then the clock ticks loudly with a menacing quality. Clearly, if the surgery is already running late, or the doctor is tired, it is going to be even more difficult to allow more time to a difficult or upsetting patient.

Strategies for managing time

Our agonised obsession with the hourglass has resulted in a good deal of discussion about time management in general practice. The subject features in books written to help doctors to avoid 'stress' and there are even courses that doctors can go on to learn how to manage their time. What strategies are available for the doctor faced by a patient who is clearly going to need more than the average 10 minutes?

Should we say we cannot deal with a big emotional problem today and ask the patient to come back tomorrow? This is not usually a good idea, because the patient may be just at the point where his need to be heard has become critical. He may have been trying to get up courage for some time, he may have been waiting several days already for an appointment with the doctor he knows and trusts. Something already said in the consultation may have released some deep feelings and made the tears start to flow. So it is better to sit back and listen and give the patient at least another 10 minutes. After that, when he or she is almost certainly beginning to feel better, it is possible gently to close the first instalment of the consultation and invite the patient back within a short time. These days, with a computer on every desk, it is possible for the doctor to book the appointment personally before the patient leaves the room. This gives a powerful message to the patient that the doctor is really interested in continuing the dialogue and the relationship. We can also offer a double appointment a few days in advance before all the slots are filled.

Will a subsequent double appointment be enough? Do some patients deserve more of the doctor's time because of the depth or nature of their distress? What about a special long appointment, out of surgery hours? There is a great fear that we may encourage some patients to become 'too dependent' on us if we are too generous with our time. In the early days of Balint groups, GP members were encouraged to invite their difficult patients for an hour-long consultation with the aim of getting to know them better. This was so much the expectation that the GPs in Michael Balint's groups would not even dare to present a patient unless they had already done this. Later, Balint and his GP colleagues came to see the long interview as 'a foreign body' in general practice. They switched their attention to what could be done in the short consultations of everyday general practice. How long would those consultations be? We are back to '6 minutes for the patient'. But Balint had realised that he should not be asking his GP colleagues to become psychotherapists. To do that they would have to leave general practice which would defeat the object of the endeavour. What they needed was to become emotionally sensitised family doctors, aware of the transcendent importance of the ever-present doctor–patient relationship.

Nevertheless, there is still an important place in general practice for the single long consultation, lasting about three-quarters of an hour and taking place at a planned time out of surgery hours:

A woman of 29 consulted the doctor frequently about pains in the back and legs, tiredness, headaches and irregular periods. She was referred to a rheumatologist and a gynaecologist. Her pains failed to improve significantly with physiotherapy. Then she and her husband of 1 year came and told the doctor that she was 'fainting' or almost passing out several times a day and suffering from giddiness. She said she felt that life was passing her by and admitted that she had had an unhappy childhood. She agreed to come for a long session after surgery. At this consultation she described how her father (whom she adored) had died when she was 14. After that life was never the same. She felt that her mother was indifferent to her and the family arranged a marriage with a man who physically abused her. She had run away and managed to obtain a divorce. She loved her present husband who was good to her but he found her ill health bewildering and she felt jealous of him if he spoke to other women. After this consultation, she continued to have back and leg pain but no longer had fainting episodes or complained of headaches. She continued to see the doctor quite regularly for consultations of normal length but the relationship was different. She was less demanding and he felt that she trusted him to look after her.

This sort of special session can obviously only be done on an occasional basis but it can be very helpful. It is perhaps most helpful for clarifying the needs of patients with multiple physical symptoms. Some people with painful past histories will need more time and can be referred to the counsellor or the local department of psychology or psychotherapy.

Conclusion

If we are able to keep calm and not let time frighten us too much, there are a number of options for managing it in ways which will satisfy our patients without damaging our own health. It is important to let the patient have sufficient time in the immediate 'crisis' situation to feel that he has been heard and recognised. Then arrangements can be made for a follow-up consultation when it is relatively convenient. If there is a torrential outpouring of pent up feelings, we must just take a deep breath, offer the tissues, sit back and let the day be ruined. And if we still experience feelings of panic when the surgery is running late, it is worth remembering that it may be a reflection of the way we feel about the person currently occupying the patient's chair.

References

1   Marvell A (1972) To his coy mistress. In: H Gardner (ed) *New Oxford Book of English Verse*. Oxford University Press, Oxford.

2   Balint E and Norell J (eds) (1973) *Six Minutes for the Patient: interactions in general practice consultation*. Tavistock Publications, London.

3   Morell DC, Evans ME, Morris RW, Roland MO (1986) The 'five minute' consultation: effect of time constraint on clinical content and patient satisfaction. *BMJ*. **292**: 870–3.

11

What are you feeling, doctor? Group members reflect on their experience

John Salinsky

The members of our research group met together regularly over a period of 5 years. At the end of this period, and towards the end of the writing of this book, I wanted to explore with the group members the ways in which they felt that the experience of the group had affected them. Had they changed in any perceptible way as people? Had they learned anything from our discussions which had altered the way they practised? There were only 10 people in the group, including the two leaders. How could any change in their work be detected or measured? How could I measure personality change? Should I make use of some established questionnaires or rating scales? Should I develop my own? Should I be searching out the group members' patients to see if they were enjoying the benefits of better understanding, sharper diagnosis, more compassionate and skilful management?

All these approaches seemed to be obstructed by a dense undergrowth of confounding factors. Any method of enquiry which involves simple counting or percentages or mean positions on a sliding scale seems to be doomed to failure when applied to complex human variables. The outcome is likely to be all the more disappointing if the number of subjects is small and statistical power quite puny. So, I decided to avoid trying to measure change in the members of the research group in any quantitative way.

Instead I decided to make use of some of the methods of qualitative research. In this approach[1-3] the researcher is able to collect data in a much more inclusive way. He can talk to any person or observe any group of people who might be able to illuminate the general area to which his curiosity has taken him. As the data collection progresses, the observer's curiosity begins to interact with his findings. He becomes aware of puzzles or contradictions and new phenomena not previously thought about. He is able to include new questions as the data collection proceeds. Themes and threads emerge from what he hears and experiences and this enables him to construct theories to explain what is going on. These ideas can then be reviewed with colleagues and by personal reflection. Further thoughts are generated and these can be checked out by further interviews with the subjects. The search for meaning can be pursued to wherever the trail seems to lead.

Qualitative research does not produce powerful statistical predictions about the extent to which a clinical intervention will save lives or reduce morbidity. But it does provide a way of searching for meaning and change in subtle and complex human interactions. Which brings us back to the doctor–patient relationship.

For a short time I considered the possibility of using the group members' patients as my research subjects. It would be really interesting, I thought, to talk to some of the patients who knew their doctors well to see if they had been aware of any changes during the period in which the research group was running. However, the practical problems, especially the proper selection of patients, seemed very daunting, and there was also the ethical problem of invading the privacy of the patient's relationship with his doctor and inevitably stirring things up. I regretfully abandoned the idea of interviewing patients but it remains on top of a filing cabinet in the inner office of my mind, waiting to be picked up one day.

Doing the research: collecting and assessing the data

For the present I decided to interview all the members of the group, including the two leaders, to see if I could discover in what ways they might have changed as a result of 5 years of regular case presentation and discussion in our group. I interviewed each person for about 15 minutes, recording the interview on a portable cassette recorder. Another member of the group interviewed me in a similar way. Most of the recordings were made in people's homes, including my own. I also carried out a group interview or 'focus group' session in which the group as a whole were invited to discuss some of the issues raised by the individual interviews. The interviews were very short compared with standard practice in qualitative research but I had been close to all the respondents for a long time and the interview was only the culmination of years of conversation about the doctor–patient relationship. I found it quite easy to write detailed notes of the interviews while listening to the tapes, so I decided not to have them professionally transcribed. By listening to the tapes several times I was able to fill in any gaps in my notes and correct the mistakes. Interviewing and transcribing was followed by an editing process in which I underlined what I saw as possibly significant themes or categories in the material. I also looked for themes or ideas which recurred or were echoed in several of the interviews. After this I tried to group the main ideas and reduce them to a smaller number of unifying or underlying themes. Qualitative research is essentially a circular process in which the researcher collects material, orders it, reflects on the meaning, makes some tentative hypotheses and then returns to 'the field' to ask more questions. In this way it is possible to follow interesting leads to a greater depth or check out puzzles and contradictions. The first 'account' can then be refined and modified and the circular process repeated, ideally until the sources yield no more new, enlightening or clarifying information.

The background: the group and its members

Before we look at some of the material produced by the interviews it might be helpful to be reminded of the composition of the group and its pattern of meeting. There were 10 of us altogether including our two leaders. Six were men and four were women. We were all GPs, although one of us had retired from active practice. Our ages ranged from late 30s to early 70s. Two of the older members had retired from being GP principals but were still seeing patients regularly as locums. Two more would reach their planned retirement age about a year after the group finished meeting. So we were a fairly seasoned bunch of family doctors and all of us had spent many years in Balint groups of one sort or another. Four of us had been in groups with Michael Balint himself and eight had taken part in previous research groups with Enid Balint. We had all led groups ourselves, mainly in the context of GP vocational training schemes. None of us had had any formal training in psychology or psychotherapy although some of us had experienced personal analysis.

The rhythm of the group's meetings was unusual in that we met for a whole day (either Saturday or Sunday) at intervals of 2–3 months during the 5-year period. We all knew each other extremely well because our common interests in Balint work and general practice education were constantly bringing us together. All these background factors may have a bearing on the ways in which the experience in the group might have enabled its members to change the way they worked, the way they felt and the way they were.

What did I want to find out?

I started off the enquiry wanting to know if and how the group members had changed. But what did I understand by the word 'change'? Michael Balint[4] famously said that work in a Balint group could lead to 'a small though significant change in personality'. I do not think this meant that people would become temperamentally different so that their friends would say, 'What has come over you? You used to be so cheerful (or impatient or self-obsessed or whatever)'. I think he meant that the acquisition of a little bit of insight about our own emotional reactions would represent a very subtle modification of the self. However, and this is the 'significant' part, such insights might make a substantial difference to the way we behaved and felt with our patients. In other words, a small change in the personal self might have a significant effect on the professional part of the self and the way we do our job. I wanted to find out whether any 'insights' gained from the group discussions had actually been translated into a different approach, a different attitude to the patient in the surgery. Even without conscious insight, I thought it was possible that the impact of the group experience at an unconscious level might lead to changes in behaviour. I also wanted to know in what ways being in this group had felt different from previous groups, because there was an impression from our conversations in the group that many people felt that we had 'gone further' than previous groups had taken them.

The starter questions

In each of my interviews I used the same little group of 'starter questions' whose purpose was to get the subject talking and thinking about the area in which I was chiefly interested. If there was a digression I could use one of the questions to bring the conversation back to what I regarded as the central focus. These were the questions.

1   Thinking about the time you spent in the research group, do you feel that your approach to patients has changed in any way?

2   Thinking of the patients you presented, has your attitude to them and the way you have interacted with them changed in any way as a result of the discussion in the group?

3   Have you come across any similar patients with whom you have been able to modify your defences?

4   In the group we talked about 'warning lights' that told us when a defence was about to operate. Did you discover any personal warning lights?

5   Did you feel that this group was different from other Balint groups you had been in?

Results

After responding to the starter questions, the group members talked quite freely about their thoughts and feelings. A number of themes emerged associated with the areas of discussion loosely defined by the questions.

Reflecting on how their approach to patients might have changed, a number of people said that they had not really changed fundamentally. Perhaps they were too old to change. On the other hand they might have been undergoing gradual change simply as a result of getting 'older and wiser'.

Listening to patients

A number of people spoke about a change in the way they listened to patients. They seemed to be listening more closely without needing to interrupt the patient. There was an increase in self-reflection. While listening to the patient they were also listening to themselves. *Stay with the pain*, one doctor now says to himself. *Whatever's going on, don't be deflected.* Several group members said that they were much more aware of their own emotional reactions to what the patient was saying. *It aroused my curiosity about my own reactions. As they are talking I think: why am I reacting like this?* This awareness helped one doctor to avoid getting into arguments or even 'blazing rows' with patients. Often there was a feeling of wanting to dictate to the patient, tell him what to do, tell him that his beliefs were totally misconceived. (This corresponds very closely to Balint's 'apostolic function' in which the doctor feels a powerful need to impose his own values on the patient.) As a result of the group experience, the doctors seemed to feel that they were able to free themselves from the apostolic function. They might not agree with the patient's views but they were able to hear him out and show that they appreciated the emotional charge behind some of these 'misguided' beliefs. This seems to imply a greater acceptance and tolerance of patients' feelings. *I'm not so frustrated with people who are ignorant or have crazy ideas. I like to find out why they are so passionate about it. If they can see that I accept their anxiety it may help them to agree in the end (e.g. that a vaccine is desirable).* Or in the words of another doctor: 'You can't force your will on people however right you are. If you take a laid back approach, sometimes they come round'. In *The Doctor, His Patient and the Illness*,[4] Michael Balint wrote that, 'The ability to listen is a new skill' for family doctors trained in conventional history taking by interrogation. 'In learning to listen to patients', he says, 'the doctor begins to listen in the same way to himself'. We are not surprised to learn that he thinks that learning to listen properly requires 'a limited though considerable change in personality'. What might surprise us is that the doctors studied here, who had spent half a lifetime in Balint groups, were only just beginning to reap the benefits of learning how to listen to their patients and themselves. Was there something different about the research group that enabled them to make a belated but significant advance in emotional awareness? I shall return to this question later.

Individual insights and lessons

A number of group members said that they had realised something specific about themselves which had enabled them to make alterations in their way of relating to patients.

Doctor B observed that it was very unusual for her to be upset by, or to fall out with, a patient. This was in marked contrast to some of the other group members who seemed frequently to feel outraged by their patients and have unpleasant confrontational scenes with them. She had begun to feel that her relationships with some patients were a little too 'cosy and comfortable' because she did not want to risk 'rocking the boat'. On a recent occasion, after the group had finished presenting new cases, she had discussed with the practice counsellor one of these collusive relationships and this had been helpful. *I think my defences against being upset are firmly in place but I've identified a problem that I have.*

Doctor C felt he had become much more aware of how close he was to patients, how important they were to him. This was partly due to the fact that he was due to retire shortly. There was a sense of imminent loss *but I don't think I would have been so aware if I hadn't been in this group.* He thought that he had become much too involved with one of the patients he had presented and was now trying to distance himself and involve other members of the practice team.

Doctor F felt that she had been 'reprimanded' by the group in the discussion on one of her cases. She had realised that she would sometimes become very negative towards a patient with a demand that she found unacceptable (such as a request for sleeping tablets). She now found that she was able to listen to what the patient had to say and explore his feelings about needing the medication. *I let myself listen and reflect in most cases. I involve myself in a bit of discussion. I still say 'no' in most cases but I feel more comfortable. Before, I thought I was doing it quite well – very open and honest. The group made me realise that I can still be honest and decline – but there is a nicer way.*

In my own interview, I said that I thought that my way of being with old ladies had changed as a result of my presentation of the 'lady with the hearing aid' case and the subsequent discussion. I was less likely to feel irritated with old ladies. I realised that they sometimes reminded me of my own elderly mother. I was now more often able to tell myself that they couldn't help being deaf, or cognitively impaired, and that it was worth making an effort to be kind and patient. It has actually become easier to be kind and patient.

Warning lights

During our discussions in the group we frequently spoke about 'warning lights' which might provide us with a useful signal that an unnecessary and counter-productive defence mechanism was about to click into place. Sometimes the lights were red and sometimes they were amber but they were always warnings of danger ahead. We thought it would be useful both to ourselves and to other doctors who had not been in a research group to be able to identify warning lights. If they were recognised in time it might be possible to slow down, reflect on what was happening and at least modify the defences so that they were less destructive.

In the interviews, some doctors were able to identify situations which in themselves turned on the warning light or made it more likely to show. Patients who presented themselves as 'emergencies' were likely to incur the doctor's anger if there was no blood to be seen. Patients with strongly held health beliefs which the doctor considered absurd and unscientific could also arouse a doctor's anger. After the group, the appearance of these patients in the surgery was enough to warn some doctors that aggressive defences (pre-emptive strikes?) were about to be deployed.

Sometimes doctors noticed that they would interrupt a patient's discourse with an abrupt change from listening to physical examination. We realised that this was likely to happen if the patient's story was arousing intolerable emotions in the doctor. One doctor found that a warning light for him when this was about to happen was: *I'm aware of a feeling that I should be doing something. I might reach for the blood pressure cuff. Am I running away from whatever is going on here and trying to stop the patient in some way? And then I don't act. I concentrate on what's going on.* This doctor had been particularly shocked on one occasion when he had stood up to apply the blood pressure cuff and had noticed for the first time that the patient was crying (*see* Chapter 8).

Another doctor said that the warning was not so much a light as a *physical barrier. So powerful. Like a steel shutter coming down. When I see that happening I try to relax a bit. Whereas before I would just go blindly on.* The most significant warning sign for this doctor was *when I want to take them by the shoulders and tell them to 'take the medicine!' or 'do what I say!'.*

Frequently, doctors said that, once they had become aware of the light on the mental dashboard, they had been able to relax and to dispel some of the tension they realised they were feeling. There were a number of physical manifestations of this tension such as: *I can feel the heat growing under my collar. That's a warning that I'm going to react and say something I will regret.* Another physical warning was: *I'm on the verge of being impatient when I'm aware of feeling a bit tight inside. 'Oh dear, this is going to go on for ever' ... a bit knotted in there.*

Did recognition of warning lights prove helpful? On many occasions it did. One doctor (Dr F) said: 'I immediately see the group in the room. With the mind's eye, I see the transcript. I sit up and say to myself: "Now you've got to behave!"'. This immediately enabled her to prevent herself from reacting in a hostile way to a patient making unacceptable demands. Another doctor on feeling the warning sign will try not to respond emotionally but say: *Let me think about what you are saying a bit more deeply,* or something like that. My own response to a feeling of irritation was *awareness that danger lay that way. There was another way that led to a pleasanter part of my personality.*

Follow-up of patients

On the whole the further information which the group members were able give me about the patients they had presented was disappointingly sparse. A number of the patients described at length in this book had left the district or had not been seen again. One elderly patient had died. The doctors told me about some patients who had not been used as cases in the book, but there were no very remarkable developments. My impression is that the lessons learned in the group had been a bit too late for the presented patients but there is evidence from the interviews documented above that a later group of patients were able to benefit from some of the increased self-awareness of the doctors.

Interviewing the group leaders

The leaders had not presented cases themselves and so were less able to comment on changes in themselves. However, both had reflected on their own practice and past history of relationships with patients. Both thought that there had been a change in the mode of presenting cases in the course of time. *The angle of approach has changed. They come at the patient from a slightly different angle. One thinks of a circle. Not from the east but from east-south-east. It makes a difference. Not so head on.*

Both leaders agreed that the group members had made some advances in spite of the fact that they were already very experienced GPs. *I think that they almost all realised something about themselves that they didn't start out with. There was a degree of openness and courage. Much greater than we have experienced previously.*

Was this group different from all other groups?

Everyone, including the leaders, said that it was different. It was longer in duration than previous groups most people had experienced. Everyone knew each other very well and the membership was constant. There were no 'strangers' in the group. *There was no one I didn't trust.* All these factors helped to create a climate in which it felt safe for members to look at their difficulties and their mistakes. It was also the only Balint group anyone had experienced in which looking at factors in one's personal history was actually encouraged. The Balint tradition has always been to discourage any exploration of the resonance between feelings induced by the patient's distress and any current problems or past grief which the doctor might carry in his or her 'personal self'. *I was never allowed (in a previous group) to discuss patients who were a particular hang-up for me or others. The leader wouldn't allow it and some of the doctors didn't like it.* In the research group no one was pressured into making personal revelations. But we were encouraged by each other to consider whether any personal factors might be operating. Perhaps the key question was: 'Would this have upset other doctors?' And if not, 'I wonder why it upset me?' We said, 'What about it? Would you like to say something?' It was an invitation not to back off. And another member said: 'In previous groups I have identified problems in myself. The difference here was that we could work on it with the group'.

Should we have had a psychoanalyst?

One member said he felt some regret that the group did not have a psychoanalyst as one of the leaders. *I felt uneasy about this. I didn't know what a psychoanalyst would have said. Would he find glaring things we hadn't thought of? It would be nice to have that part (transference) looked at by someone who is used to dealing with these issues.* When I put this question to other group members, the general view was that, with a psychoanalyst, the group would have been different and perhaps would have been unable to achieve the kind of things it did achieve. It would have been interesting but it would have been a different kind of group.

Conclusions

Group members felt they had gained in the following ways:

- an improved ability to listen to patients;

- an enhanced awareness of one's own feelings while listening;

- a greater willingness to suspend one's own 'apostolic' agenda and let the patient continue with his. Instead of interrupting, the doctors now felt they were trying to understand why a patient's ideas were so important to him;

- a greater willingness to accept and tolerate patients' feelings and ideas, however 'misguided' they seem to the doctor;

- identifying some of one's own individual problems in handling emotion in the consultation;

- recognising personal 'warning lights' which enable one to disengage or modify defences which are unhelpful.

The research group had enabled these gains to be made because it was a safe place in which to work. Everyone was known and trusted. Group members felt free to reflect on the reasons why certain types of patient always made them go on the defensive. In some cases these reflections involved quite personal and private matters. It was possible to discuss and explore these issues in the group in a way that the doctors had not previously experienced in a Balint group.

During the group interview, Michael Courtenay said at one point: 'I have a feeling that we have pushed a little door ajar which had always been tight shut because of the contract that the Balints initially put out. I think that pressure has built up in us over the years to need to open this door, very gingerly, not very far, rather fearful of what was going to be on the other side. And when we did so we found the light was on – next door ...'. And Erica Jones added: 'Even if it was only a 40 watt bulb!'

I would like to thank Richard Addison PhD, Associate Clinical Professor in the Department of Family and Community Medicine, University of California School of Medicine, San Francisco for his advice and help with the design of the study and the writing of this chapter.

References

1 Crabtree BF, Miller WL (eds) (1999) *Doing Qualitative Research*, 2e. Sage Publications, Thousand Oaks, CA.

2 Packer MJ, Addison RB (eds) (1989) *Entering the Circle: hermeneutic investigation in psychology*. State University of New York Press, Albany NY.

3 Gantley M, Harding G, Kumar S, Tissier J (1999) *Master Classes in Primary Care Research No 1: an introduction to qualitative methods for health professionals*. Royal College of General Practitioners, London.

4 Balint M (1957) *The Doctor, His Patient and the Illness*. Pitman, London. 2e, 1964; Millennium edition, 2000. Churchill Livingstone, Edinburgh.

12

What can doctors do?

In earlier chapters we have given examples of what can happen when a family doctor is unable to cope with empathic sharing of a patient's emotions and withdraws to a safe distance. Sometimes this is necessary for the doctor's emotional wellbeing – there is a limit to the amount of other people's pain which any of us can bear. On the other hand, there are many occasions when the reaction away from the patient's feelings is too sudden and violent – out of proportion to the amount of pain which we might experience. When this happens there is a loss, maybe a serious loss, for the patient which both doctor and patient will regret.

We have already discussed Tom Main's paper[1] in which he suggested that family doctors might try to learn to tailor their 'defences' a little more exactly to the requirements of each case. This would involve gaining sufficient insight into the reasons for our reactions to enable us to slow things down, modify our instant responses, creep back out of our shells (when it's safe to do so) and bravely re-engage with the patient.

How are we to go about this process of rationalising our responses to patients' emotions? We are clearly going to need a heightened awareness of everything that is going on in the patient, in ourselves and in the environment which might be relevant.

Predisposing factors

To start with, we know that there are a number of predisposing factors which will make us more likely to avoid subjective encounters with our patients' feelings. These have already been discussed in Chapter 9. They include tiredness, illness, preoccupation with personal problems, anger with colleagues in the practice team and oppression by shortage of time. Perhaps the word 'stress' sums it all up and plenty of serious attention has been given in recent years to the problem of anticipating stress and its dreaded sequel 'burnout' among professionals.[2,3] Doctors, and indeed all health workers, need to do all they can they to create working conditions for themselves in which external stress is minimised. Equally obviously, our success in this worthwhile endeavour will be limited. There are still going to be times when we let down a patient who needs us to be present emotionally – simply because we are exhausted and debilitated. The important thing is to be aware that when we are under stress these undesirable things may happen and we should try very hard not to let them happen with those needy patients. If the consultation still goes wrong there may be possibilities of rescue, as we shall describe later.

Warning lights

However, even when we are not under stress, a consultation can easily suffer from emotional deprivation for other reasons to do with the doctor and/or the patient. We know from these cases that events happen very quickly where emotional self-protection is concerned. Within seconds of the doctor's perception of danger the personal self can be tightly rolled up in a ball with a prickly exterior. Fortunately there are some warning signs that this is going to happen. Red or amber lights can be clearly seen once we know what to look out for. Sensing them requires us to monitor both our feelings and our behaviour in the very early stages of the consultation. Some patients will induce in a previously calm and benign doctor all sorts of negative feelings. Free-floating anxiety is an important one to recognise. More specifically, the doctor may notice restlessness and irritability as a response to the patient's opening gambit or even the way he looks as he enters the room. The man who wanted sleeping pills (Chapter 2) aroused irritation first by his appearance and his entrance (preceding the doctor) and then by his unacceptable request. A nervous look at the clock or an inner voice which wails: 'This is going to take too long, I can't cope with this now' can be another warning sign. It may be the wavelength of the emotional signals coming from the patient (e.g. the lady with the hearing aid in Chapter 3) rather than the lateness of the hour which sounds the alarm about 'not enough time'.

Some patients immediately make us feel angry, perhaps in response to the patient's anger, whether expressed or quietly seething. If we allow ourselves to respond angrily, a battle is soon raging. The fight may provide both participants with some enjoyment but all chance of reaching mutual understanding will be (temporarily) lost. Alternatively, we may start going out of our way to be ingratiating and to avoid any conflict with someone who actually makes us feel angry. The consultation will then be superficially friendly but lacking in real engagement.

Patients who are also colleagues may give rise to defensive behaviour as we discovered from the case of the doctor whose patient was also his health visitor (Chapter 1). Here it was difficult for the doctor to accept that a competent, helpful and supportive member of his team could also be a frightened patient needing to be held emotionally herself.

A feeling of coolness and contempt for a patient who seems stupid and pathetic may be another warning to be aware of. We know we are normally kind and considerate to someone who is struggling. Perhaps this person stutters and stumbles in a way which is all too familiar from our own personal struggles. We don't want to get too close to that weakness and contempt puts us safely on the safe side with the bullies. The hearing aid lady comes to mind again. This sort of self-knowledge will almost certainly not come until much later, if it comes at all. The important preventive measure is to recognise the feeling as a warning sign; a sign that empathy is greatly needed and it has just flown out of the window.

Defensive strategies

On other occasions we may use more subtle defensive strategies. Our behaviour with the patient may be perfectly reasonable and in accordance with all the best guidelines and recommendations. We may decide to ignore the patient's personality and concentrate on his body, telling ourselves that this, after all, is what we have been trained to do. The methodical routine of the clinical examination can be very soothing. It can serve as a displacement activity to divert energy away from distressed or angry feelings about the owner of the body being examined. When we address the owner as a person again we simply report on our clinical findings. Any signs of organic illness will lead the conversation safely on towards blood tests, X-rays, referrals and prescriptions. All this activity may be perfectly appropriate. However, when the initial consultation has been difficult and the relationship prickly, we should ask ourselves whether we are doing it mainly to avoid contact with the patient's feelings; and, of course, we might be trying to suppress the arousal of our own feelings.

Sometimes we may decide that the safest way to relate to a patient is not to listen to him talking about how he feels but to give him some sound advice. We are, after all, physicians and we need to educate our woefully ignorant clients. The doctor knows best and the patient would do well to pay attention! Of course, health education is a perfectly appropriate and necessary part of our work (although nurses may do it better) but we need to be careful of any overzealous 'apostolic function'. We should listen out for the sound we make when we are giving a health education lecture and check that we are not using it as a way of dealing with emotional discomfort. The underlying, semiconscious motive might be: 'I don't want to hear any more about this man's misery. It's clear that he needs to go on a diet and get more exercise so I shall lay that out for him as plainly as I can. Then, of course, it's up to him'.

A similar situation occurs when the patient refuses to take the medication, or gets the tablets muddled and uses the antibiotic for pain relief or to get to sleep. We don't want to engage with his incomprehensible feelings about the medicine as this may provoke irritation (as in the case of the lady in Chapter 5 who wouldn't take her thyroxine) and so we become very cool and reasonable. We do the best we can in the face of invincible ignorance.

'Practice policies' can also be used to hide behind when the emotional temperature shows signs of rising to a dangerous level. If a patient turns up without an appointment and asks to be seen 'at once' and is clearly not suffering from a life-threatening condition, we may feel the need to reinforce practice policy and ask him to return another day. But it's possible that something about the patient, either in his bid for attention today or in the memory of past interactions, makes us decide that practice policy is a good way of avoiding an unwanted emotional experience. 'Rational' practice policies are also available to help us refuse certain medicines requested by the patient, such as antibiotics for presumed virus infections, sleeping tablets for those seeking temporary chemical-induced oblivion and (nowadays) any medicine the patient desires whose use is not sufficiently evidence-based. Is this behaviour rational or defensive?

Finally there is a rather different warning sign which we need to be alert to when everything in the relationship is going well. This relates to the situation in which we have become so closely identified with the patient that we cannot bear the thought of anything unpleasant happening to him. An example is the case of the patient with an apparently benign breast lump (Chapter 2) whose doctor could not consciously accept the possibility of a malignancy and so went on reassuring the patient and herself, while making every effort to get her seen quickly. We may also feel so fearful of angering the patient and thus disturbing a 'good' (but too cosy) doctor–patient relationship. We may, without realising it, become so dependent on the patient's good opinion that we are unable to say anything, however important, that might disrupt a rather superficial friendship.

The warning signs that might alert us to our defence against emotional involvement with the patient are as follows:

- anxiety;

- feeling irritable;

- worried about time;

- withdrawn and aloof;

- cold and contemptuous;

- angry;

- careful not to offend;

- overuse of the biomedical model;

- apostolic behaviour;

- health education;

- sticking firmly to practice policies;

- too closely identified.

Should all defences be abolished?

Is it always 'wrong' to be defended? Should we always engage fully with the patient's feelings even when they are being quite unreasonably demanding? Clearly there will always be some situations when defences are essential if doctors are to survive with their own emotional health intact. Some of our encounters are with people who have suffered so terribly and cruelly that even though our stony hearts are melting we need to hold back from total involvement. Some patients' sorrows may be so close to our own that it is the specificity which warns us to keep a respectful distance. In any case, there is a limit to the number of really close emotional encounters that we can cope with in the course of one day. When we sense that we are approaching the maximum safe exposure for the day our best course is to hold back a little if yet another patient bursts into tears. 'Humankind cannot bear very much reality', according to TS Eliot,[4] and doctors and health workers, being human, can only bear a limited amount of other people's reality.

Yes, we need some defences to shore us up and prevent us from being washed away. The important thing is that the defences should, as far as possible, be in proportion to the need. We should try not to shut out the patient's feelings on occasions when we could share them without too much difficulty. By sharing their feelings we would become available to our patients in a way that is helpful and healing. To make our defences appropriate we need to be able to control them and that means that they must be in the realm of consciousness, not lurking in the underworld of the unconscious. Unconscious defences spring into action very rapidly and are too quick for us to control. Before we realise consciously that one of these automatic defences is operating, the wrong things have been said, the wrong gestures made and the relationship between doctor and patient has been seriously damaged.

That is why we desperately need to know our warning signs so we can spot them like an aircraft spotter detecting approaching enemy aircraft. The characteristic signals will be different for each doctor and it is up to each of us to become familiar with our own patterns.

What can doctors do?

It should be possible for us to become aware of a few of our own warning signs in time to change course before the consultation goes wrong. Sometimes the doctor is able to change the quality of the consultation after only a brief pause. Going out of the room for a few seconds may provide sufficient breathing space for both doctor and patient to start over again. If the consultation has already started to go wrong (perhaps the patient is looking puzzled or offended) it may still not be too late.

A case history

One Saturday morning a woman brought her 16-year-old son to see the family doctor. He had a cold for the second time in a month and his mother thought he was 'run down'. She wanted an antibiotic for him and some vitamins to pick him up and improve his appetite. The doctor knew that her husband, the boy's father, had died of stomach cancer 18 months previously, that the children were having difficulty in grieving openly and the whole family had been referred for psychological help. Knowing all this background, the doctor, for some reason, still met the mother's challenge head on and told her that her son needed neither antibiotics nor extra vitamins. He ignored the warning signs (in himself) of anxiety, irritability, apostolic functioning and resorting inappropriately to health education. Perhaps the sudden appearance of the bereaved mother and son in an 'emergency' surgery set off an unconscious alarm telling him that he wouldn't be able to cope with sharing the grief and loss that was expressed indirectly in the mother's anxious concern and the son's silent, depressive posture.

The mother listened to the doctor's lecture about the body's ability to rid itself of viruses without medicines. She and the boy went away but the doctor could see that she was angry and unhappy. He remained troubled by this encounter and after the surgery he telephoned her to try and put things right. The mother reminded the doctor that her son had been iron deficient as a toddler and she told him that she felt her son needed extra vitamins to give him strength to fight off the virus. The doctor now agreed to prescribe some and offered to do some blood tests to 'make sure that he was OK'. He mentioned the loss of the husband to show her that he hadn't forgotten. Doctor and mother had a friendly conversation and she thanked him warmly for telephoning. The doctor felt much better!

This is a good example of the way in which a consultation can be 'rescued' at the last minute, or even after the patient has left the room. We should not be too proud to admit that we have made a mistake, lost control, been insensitive or lost our temper. Patients know we are not infallible but they may with good reason feel that we are unwilling to admit to human errors. As a profession we are just beginning to realise that it is a decent, helpful thing to apologise when things have gone wrong and offer to try again. There is no catastrophic loss of prestige or dignity implied. The patients appreciate our honesty and we feel better inside.

If not now, when?

If it is not possible to rescue the consultation, it may still be possible to rescue the relationship at the next consultation with the same patient. General practice is full of opportunities to have a second chance and make good one's failures. It may dawn on us at some point – on the way home, when discussing the patient with a colleague or when lying awake in bed – that a consultation failed because of inappropriate defences. It may not be too late to try again. The patient may be returning anyway or can be invited to do so to discuss some results or the possibility of referral. In a better mood, under less pressure, willing to be more accepting, we may be able to do very much better.

If there is no way of offering belated empathy to that particular patient, we can at least apply the lesson learned to the next patient or the one after that. A failure of empathy with one patient may lead us to greater awareness of important warning signs. We may well find that a particular sort of patient or problem is likely to trigger our defence mechanisms and light up the warning signs. Once we start to think of the possibility of a consultation being spoiled by an unnecessary emotional defence we are much better placed to prevent it happening.

Seeking and finding help from colleagues

All the same, this is difficult work for anyone to do entirely on their own. A doctor who has begun to realise that failure of empathy is a professional problem will be greatly helped by support from colleagues. A regular meeting can be set up within the practice at which members of the team can discuss interpersonal problems with patients. An increasing number of GPs are taking part in mentoring,[5] an arrangement in which a doctor can discuss his professional and personal development with a chosen colleague on a regular basis. Discussing a problem doctor–patient relationship with a mentor could be a very satisfactory way of learning more about why particular patients arouse unhelpful defences.

At present, mentoring is an optional facility which GPs have to seek out for themselves. Counsellors and social workers, on the other hand, work in a culture where supervision is provided for everyone by senior members of the profession. Family doctors are just as acutely exposed to powerful emotions but they are expected to work without the safety net of supervision. Perhaps the time has come for us to provide mentoring or supervision for all doctors as a basic necessity.

Balint groups

Finally, since this was the setting of our work on the subject, we must return to the Balint group. A doctor who is interested in improving his awareness of the emotions in the consultation might well benefit from joining an ongoing group. Such a group, meeting every week or two, is able to listen to presentations of each of its members' problems and provide eight or nine different views of what is going on in the relationship. As the members of the group get to know one another they begin to feel safer in the group and it becomes easier to admit one's stupidities and some of one's more personal thoughts and feelings.

Unfortunately there is a difficulty finding a group to join. There are a number of reasons for this shortage. Balint groups were originally always led by psychoanalysts and, although this is no longer the case, there is still a shortage of GPs with sufficient experience (and confidence) to lead a group. Groups do need some leadership if they are to stay focused on the work and remain a secure and safe place in which to confide one's feelings. Groups also need members and, although Michael Balint's work is widely known and respected, GPs have never rushed to join groups in large numbers. Shortage of time has always been the difficulty – especially as a group requires a weekly or fortnightly commitment for several years if it is to reap the benefits of its maturity. Now, of course, groaning under our new contracts and our healthcare planning responsibilities, we have even less time. But perhaps a greater consciousness of the need to understand the emotional dimension of our work with patients might induce more doctors to find time for an activity with a high priority.

Training – or treatment?

We have looked at ways in which doctors might train themselves to become more aware of 'warning lights' and become less defensive than they might be, or need to be. Working with a mentor or in a group is likely to enhance self-awareness in the consultation. But is 'training' going to be sufficient? How far can one learn in this way to be more open, less evasive, less afraid? What if some of the problems go right down to the depths of our own personalities: to the experiences, the feelings, the conflicts which have made us who we are? Do doctors themselves need therapy if they are to solve the problem of their own counterproductive defences?

Ever since Balint groups started, there has been heated discussion about whether they could or should be considered as a form of psychotherapy for the participants. Balint himself described the business of his groups as 'training-cum-research'. He was careful to point out that the groups were not there to provide 'therapy'. Applicants to the early groups were screened to exclude the seriously unbalanced (reasonably enough) and also those who might, misguidedly, see the group as an opportunity for personal treatment. Why was he so particular about this? Essentially, because the groups were intended to focus on the doctor–patient relationship and to be primarily of benefit to patients. The majority of group members had enlisted because they wanted to learn more about the psychological aspects of general practice and not because they wanted personal therapy. Many people who might benefit from the less intrusive, patient-centred approach would be put off. Potential newcomers would be scared that they might be subjected to interrogations about their childhood, their sexual history, and their most personal and private feelings. Ironically, despite the Balints' strict and watchful avoidance of this kind of thing, this was exactly the kind of reputation that Balint groups had for many doctors who had no personal experience of them. It did the movement a great deal of harm and prevented Balint groups from being regarded as part of mainstream medical education until relatively recently.

Today, Balint groups are used in some vocational training programmes in this country, in Europe and the USA. There are also still groups for mature practitioners although, as we have seen, not many in the UK. The groups aim to help their members towards a better understanding of the emotional elements in the doctor–patient relationship and hence to achieve better all-round patient care. The group leaders do not offer therapy but they might well hope for some change of attitude in the participants in the course of a period of 1 to 3 years. This would correspond to Michael Balint's 'limited but considerable change in personality'. This rather teasing phrase has puzzled students of Balint for many years. 'Considerable' sounds quite substantial but 'limited' sounds unimpressive. Were the Balints really aiming to provide therapy artfully disguised as 'training'? On one occasion, Michael Balint was heard to make a rather revealing 'Freudian' slip. When asked how long a doctor would need to be in a group to achieve some benefit from it he said: 'It takes about 2 years of treatment – I mean training'.[6]

It is difficult to prove that Balint training for doctors improves the quality of care for their patients. All one can say is that those who have joined a group and stayed the course for 3 or 4 years will generally say that it opened their eyes and gave them a way of thinking about the interplay of feelings in the consulting room which has been of lasting value.

However, there will be some doctors who feel that, for them, reflection with a supervisor or participation in a group is not sufficient. They may have begun to discover things about their own inner world and their own emotional development which are troubling them. Personal therapy of one sort or another would then be the next step, particularly for those who feel that their professional and personal functioning is showing signs of serious dysfunction.

Personal therapy is not part of the training curriculum for family doctors as it is for counsellors and psychotherapists, although some might argue that it should be. Under present conditions the majority of doctors are not going to consider it. But some sort of training in reflection and self-awareness would be worthwhile for everyone. A Balint group is only one possible option. There are many opportunities every day in the surgery to examine the emotional content of our consultations. On our own or with the help of colleagues, with a partner, a tutor, a mentor or a group, we can reflect on those encounters which have gone wrong or failed to achieve their potential because of unnecessary or inappropriate withholding of empathy on the part of the doctor.

We can learn to recognise the warning signs and gradually increase our insight into our own reactions.

References

1   Main T (1978) Some medical defences against involvement with patients. *J Balint Soc*. **7**: 3–11.

2   Rout U, Rout JK (1993) *Stress and General Practitioners*. Kluwer Medical, Dordrecht.

3   Haslam D (ed) (2000) *Not Another Guide to Stress in General Practice!* (2e). Radcliffe Medical Press, Oxford.

4   Eliot TS (1941) Burnt Norton. In: *Four Quartets*. Faber and Faber, London.

5   Freeman R (1998) *Mentoring in General Practice*. Butterworth Heinemann, Oxford.

6   Courtenay MJF (1998) Personal communication.

13

Implications for medical education

Case history

A medical student in the 1960s was looking after a 50-year-old man who had suffered a myocardial infarct. In those days the patient was treated with fairly prolonged bed rest and the student saw him briefly on most days. He would ask how he was and make some reassuring remark about his treatment and prognosis. The patient wasn't very talkative and about all the student knew about him was that he was married and had a son aged 10. One day the patient suddenly asked when he would be able to resume sexual intercourse. The student was extremely embarrassed but said he would try and find out the answer. Fortunately, he was about to attend his first Balint seminar, run at that time by Michael Balint himself. The student was diffident about presenting the case since he knew so little about the patient, but eventually plucked up the courage to do so. Balint encouraged the group to speculate about what might be going on and the student soon realised that he knew a good deal more about the man than he thought. The group came up with ideas which might have been relevant, such as that the man worked abroad a lot, had married late and only had one son. Could he be eager to please women other than his wife? Might his sexual performance be a lot more important to him than at first seemed to be the case? The student felt in a position to go back and understand his patient

> better. At the same time Balint urged the group to look out the literature on sexual intercourse after myocardial infarction, an early example of the evidence-based approach.

This example crystallises many of the aims of medical training laid down by the General Medical Council (GMC).[1] It was important for the student to learn about, among other things:

• the diagnosis of the medical condition;

• its investigation and management;

• the implications of this potentially fatal illness;

• its effect on the patient;

• the ideas and concerns of this particular patient;

• the prognosis of the illness;

• its management after discharge from hospital;

• the impact of the case on the student;

• the importance of striving for high standards of care.

The GMC document *Tomorrow's Doctors* lists the knowledge, skills and attitudes that students should acquire during their undergraduate medical education. The authors point out the two essential aims of this period of education. These are to prepare for the house officer year and to prepare for lifelong practice. To fulfil the first aim requires the student to concentrate on understanding matters of immediate application. To fulfil the second aim requires a flexibility that has often been lacking in undergraduate curricula. The GMC now recommends that the curriculum includes learning to help students deal with the 'unforeseeable' situations that they are certain to meet during their practising lifetimes.

How are these broader aims and more specific objectives, such as those listed above, being met at the moment? It appears that, following the GMC recommendations, a very slow and painful process of change in undergraduate education began. It is now customary, for example, for students to have contact with patients at an early stage of their education and some medical schools have succeeded in integrating preclinical and clinical education. While rote learning and curriculum cramming are far from eliminated, there is a welcome move towards discovery learning and towards dealing with principles rather than facts.

When it comes to vocational training for general practice, things appear to be getting worse rather than better. Samuel's Occasional Paper[2] offered some new ideas but in many ways it was a summary of the exciting developments that had taken place in vocational training during the previous two decades. Since then the overwhelming desire of government, perhaps reflecting society at large, has been for accountability. There has rightly been a concern for high standards and for weeding out the unacceptable but this has been at a price. The measurable has taken the place of the important. Training is in danger of superseding education. The bottom line of training is passing the very basic test of summative assessment and, for many GP registrars, anything not directly connected with passing that test is considered irrelevant.

One of the consequences of this is that the study of interpersonal issues and such matters as the doctor–patient relationship are in danger of going to the bottom of the pile. At least there is some emphasis on studying the consultation, if only so that GP regis-trars can pass their assessment of consultation skills. Pendleton and colleagues' book[3] emphasised the 'tasks' of the consultation – what had to be done and what skills should be learned to help carry out these tasks. There is now a weight of evidence that good communication within the consultation leads to better compliance, more satisfied patients, more satisfied doctors and, most impor-tant, better health outcomes. (Much of the relevant research evidence for this is discussed by Silverman and colleagues.[4])

Training in communication skills is clearly of great importance for future GPs. It helps ground them in the 'illness' model as well as the 'disease' model.[5] It allows for the rehearsal of skills which help students or GP registrars to understand the patient's perspective. It helps them to adopt a patient-centred approach to the consultation, checking out with the patient such things as the agreed agenda for the consultation, likely diagnoses and possible management options. Kurtz and colleagues[6] are leading exponents of a skills-based approach and they argue that, 'the acquisition of skills can open the path to changes in attitude'. This can often be true, but as we have seen in this book, inappropriate attitudes may well stem from strong defences. Such strong defences may prevent doctors in training from acquiring or using their new skills. It may be necessary for the trainees to be helped to acquire greater self-awareness first. Our impression is that with current methods not enough attention is paid to the doctor's own feelings. There will be occasions during consultations when the doctor knows the sort of response which is needed but he is completely unable to provide it because his own feelings are in disarray. The 'medical defences' with which he is unfamiliar will have locked into place.

Nevertheless, it is good to see that learning about the consultation has now taken centre stage in GP education. While welcoming this belated development we must be clear that the story cannot end there. There has been evidence going back many years[7,8] that, as they go through their undergraduate training, medical students become less person-centred and lose many of their humanitarian aspirations. The archaic system of junior doctor training in hospital is hardly designed to help the doctors regain their ideals. Of even greater concern is that the increasing pressures of the GP registrar year are making it more difficult for the registrars to develop the humanitarian side of their work.

We hope that the encounters discussed in this book demonstrate the important role of the doctor's personal self in GP consultations. Much of our argument is about the need for doctors to understand themselves better so that they can bring to consciousness at least some of the personal factors which prevent them from engaging in the best way with their patients. The development of this self-understanding therefore needs to occupy a central role in education. Arguably this is the first stage in what Balint[9] called 'the acquisition of psychotherapeutic skill' which, he suggested, 'inevitably entails a limited, though considerable, change in the doctor's personality'. Balint was writing in the context of seminars for established practitioners. So far as doctors in training are concerned perhaps 'personality development' is a more appropriate and acceptable phrase.

If the idea of a change in personality, or even personality development, sounds threatening, it is arguably because, at least for the past 100 years, Western medicine 'has neglected the emotions'.[10] In a lecture in 1998 McWhinney[10] quoted Crookshank writing in 1926 about the handbooks of clinical diagnosis that had appeared in the early 1900s. 'They give excellent schemes for the physical examination of the patient whilst strangely ignoring, almost completely, the psychical.' McWhinney went on to point out the absolutely central importance of listening. 'Once we learn to listen, our clinical method requires us to attend to the emotions in every case. It cannot do otherwise. We will no longer be able to live with the affect-denying clinical method that dominates our medical schools.' The emotional education of doctors has to be one of the basic themes of the educational process, informing everything else. How might we begin to provide such an education?

Perhaps the first, and most important, step is for those responsible for teaching to have the confidence to allow the learners to be exposed to highly emotional situations. So often it is our own fears, and not those of the students, that stand in the way. A pilot 2-week course at one medical school, for example, gave preclinical students an opportunity to interview a variety of patients including those in a local hospice. The organisers of the course had to fight the medical school establishment all the way. 'Talking with dying patients? How could this be appropriate or suitable for "science" students busy with anatomy and physiology?' For most of the students the experience was a moving and insightful one. 'If patients are dying, they may not necessarily be distraught. There is always a positive side', was one typical comment. 'We learnt how to cope with strong emotions, especially with terminally ill patients', was another.

Clearly, more needs to happen than merely exposing students to distraught patients. There *is* a great potential for harm if such sensitive situations are not carefully handled. On this particular course a number of methods were used from which it is possible to derive some principles for wider application:

1   The students visited the patients in pairs. This helped them to feel less exposed and isolated. It also gave them the opportunity to learn how to observe a colleague at work and to give supportive feedback.

2   The exercise was part of a 2-week course for which the students worked in small groups led by experienced facilitators. Thus, a climate of safety was established from which the group members could move on to more challenging tasks, though always in a supportive environment. Baldwin and Williams[11] describe this process in some detail, emphasising the need for a 'series of steps, each dependent on the previous one being completed, in an incremental development of challenge and support'.

3   There was the opportunity for each student to have an individual review from one of the facilitators at least once during the course. Sometimes, a group can appear to be working well and meeting the needs of all its members but this may hide the fact that some individuals are feeling uncomfortable and insecure. The opportunity for working 1:1 is in any case important for learners to understand their individual needs and how to meet them.

4   There was a continued emphasis in the groups on supportive feedback. The 'Pendleton rules'[3] were discussed and observed. The value of such an approach to feedback is that it builds on the strengths of the learner. The feedback is based on a description of what was observed rather than on value judgements.

5   There were frequent opportunities in the groups to review both the learning process and the learning that had been achieved. The students were given the whole of the last morning of the course for a final review and this was done most creatively, with one group summarising its achievements in song. In any successful learning situation, but particularly when emotional issues are an important component, it is very easy for the participants to feel a 'rosy glow'. Later, when this feeling fades, they may be hard pressed to remember what they have learnt and so have difficulty applying it to other situations. Baldwin and

Williams[11] propose a structured way of reviewing a course that greatly enhances its learning potential:

- *recall* details of the experience;

- *reflect* about feelings at different points on the course;

- *record* details of what has been learnt;

- *review* the stage reached in terms of professional development;

- *assess* future needs.

McWhinney's[10] lecture ended with a discussion of 'listening, the essential skill'. He suggested that 'listening is at the same time a skill, a state of mind and a way of being a physician ... Without the intrusion of distracting thoughts and emotions we can respond to suffering with authentic feelings and acts of compassion. As clinicians, too, we heighten our awareness of the patient's bodily symptoms'. How are students and registrars to learn to be skilled, active listeners?

Clearly, one way is to participate in the sort of activities we have discussed in previous chapters. There is no reason, for example, why students should not take part in a mentoring programme. They may learn a lot, and feel supported, even by mentoring each other.[12] This process can be greatly helped by some initial training in mentoring of which active listening is the key component.[13,14] Greco and colleagues in Australia[15] describe an 'active listening module' in which the students work as a 'triad'. Essentially, one student is the subject and he presents a 'real' problem. The second member of the triad is the listener and the third observes. All three of the students have the opportunity to take each role. In addition a facilitator is there to 'seize every learning opportunity as it arises within the triad interaction'. The feedback offered, and the fact that the group works on 'real' situations, make this a very powerful learning experience.

We have had an illustration at the beginning of this chapter as to the value of a Balint group, at least for one student. Such a group can clearly offer enormous understanding and insight to students as well as to established doctors. Although a few GP vocational training schemes run Balint-type groups on their day-release courses, the method is still rarely used in this country. The situation is quite different in Germany. Otten[16] describes how student Balint groups work there and gives some examples of their power for enhancing the students' personal development. She also quotes some continuing research which is going some way to demonstrate the beneficial effect of attending a Balint group on doctors' consulting skills.

If Balint groups are relatively popular in Germany, in the USA humanities teaching is widely available for medical students. Studying literature in particular can enormously enrich the training of young doctors in a whole variety of ways.[17] Another very useful feature of training in the USA, as well as the widespread use of Balint groups, is the presence in each residency programme of a behavioural scientist, counsellor or similar professional.[18] They are available for consultation by the residents about patients who make them feel troubled. And is it really surprising that residents, or students, *are* troubled by their patients? Indeed we should surely be worrying if they are not, if they learn (as often appears to be the case) to repress too many of their feelings and acquire inappropriate defences. Would it not be wonderful – and only common sense – to have someone available to British medical students or junior doctors whose job it was to say, 'You all have feelings and they are going to be disturbed by patients whether you like it or not. And if you can understand your feelings you can actually use them to help patients get better'.

We hope we have succeeded in making a strong case for the central importance of emotional education in the training of doctors, particularly GPs. We have outlined a number of approaches that might be used in such an educational programme. However, there needs to be a long overdue change in attitude if this new approach is to work.

References

1   General Medical Council (1993) *Tomorrow's Doctors*. General Medical Council, London.

2   Samuel O (1990) *Towards a Curriculum for General Practice Training* (Occasional Paper 44). Royal College of General Practitioners, London.

3   Pendleton D, Schofield T, Tate P, Havelock P (1984) *The Consultation: an approach to learning and teaching.* Oxford University Press, Oxford.

4   Silverman J, Kurtz S, Draper J (1998) *Skills for Communicating with Patients.* Radcliffe Medical Press, Oxford.

5   Stewart M, Roter D (eds) (1990) *Communicating with Medical Patients.* Sage Publications, Newbury Park, CA.

6   Kurtz S, Silverman J, Draper J (1998) *Teaching and Learning Communication Skills in Medicine.* Radcliffe Medical Press, Oxford.

7   Barbee RA, Feldman SE (1970) A three year longitudinal study of the medical interview and its relationship to student performance in clinical medicine. *J Med Edu.* **45**: 770–6.

8   Preven DW, Katcher EK, Kupfer RB, Walters JA (1986) Interviewing skills in first year medical students. *J Med Edu.* **61**: 842–4.

9   Balint M (1957) *The Doctor, His Patient and the Illness.* Pitman, London. 2e, 1964; Millennium edition, 2000. Churchill Livingstone, Edinburgh.

10 McWhinney I (1999) The physician as healer: the legacy of Michael Balint. In: J Salinsky (ed) *Proceedings of the Eleventh International Balint Congress 1998.* Limited Edition Press, Southport, pp 63–71.

11 Baldwin J, Williams H (1988) *Active Learning: a trainer's guide.* Blackwell, Oxford.

12 Goodlad S (ed) (1995) *Students as Tutors and Mentors.* Kogan Page, London.

13 Freeman R (1998) *Mentoring in General Practice.* Butterworth Heinemann, Oxford.

14 Sackin P, Barnett M, Eastaugh A, Paxton P (1997) Peer-supported learning. *B J Gen Pract.* **47**: 67–8.

15 Greco M, Buckley J, Francis W (1997) Triads: an effective method for learning the art of listening. *Edu Gen Pract.* **8**: 329–34.

16 Otten H (1998) Balint work in Germany. *J Balint Soc.* **26**: 16–19.

17 Lewis P (1996) Shouldn't you read more? *Edu Gen Pract.* **7**: 306–17.

18 Salinsky J (1991) Family medicine training in the USA: any lessons for British general practice? *Postgrad Edu Gen Pract.* **2**: 187–90.

Appendix

Some medical defences against involvement with patients

Michael Balint Memorial Lecture given by Tom Main on 24 January 1978

This lecture was published in the 1978 issue of the Journal of the Balint Society. *It is reproduced here by kind permission of the Council of the Balint Society.*

After D-Day I worked at Montgomery's 21st Army Group Rear HQ as that force's senior psychiatrist, far behind the fighting. I made regular trips to and from the forward areas to make surveys about acute psychiatric casualties but could not avoid noticing the huge variations in the fighting morale of the various units. Fighting spirit and the will to win seemed to be at its lowest among troops in contact with the enemy. Unwarlike feelings were indeed quite common there, and more, were tolerated, even shared, by some junior officers; lack of zest for hardship, dislike of danger, distaste for death, bitter grief about dead comrades, resentful alienation from people leading safe lives, panic at sudden noises and so forth. None here seemed to be fired by Henry V sentiments; but the further back one went, through battalion, brigade and Divisional Headquarters, the more one could find martial favour. Fighting morale seemed to rise as the square of the distance from the enemy until, well behind the armies, at army Group Rear Headquarters, it reached its zenith. One of my seniors here was fierce that the enemy should be attacked all day and every day (by those in front of course) and as for psychiatric casualties, he wanted them all court-martialled, given a fair trial and then shot.

Your Society has invited me, a psychoanalyst and psychiatrist from the rear headquarters of specialist medicine, to address you of the medical front line. My topic is medical defences against involvement with patients, a civilian matter yet reminiscent of the front-line soldier's wish for a quiet life; a topic clearly about timidity and, at its worst, of cowardice in the face of a daunting task.

Like all from the safe rear headquarters, I find it relatively easy to recognise inaction due to cowardice in you of the medical front line; but know I am in good company. In Balint seminars with general practitioners I have often observed during discussion of a frightening and puzzling case how regularly advice is given that the case should be investigated with more vigour and courage, and how all the doctors present agree about this; except one – the coward in the front line, the doctor in charge of the case.

All analogies eventually become strained but mine can be pursued a little longer. Medicine and war are both serious with issues of life and death, crippledom and loss, sadnesses and terror about external dangers; and both are also complicated by anxieties from the inner world, unconscious fantasies of primitive sadism, punishment and so on. The front-line officer and the general practitioner is each regularly required first to contain high tensions arising from these two, inner and outer, sources and to withstand pressures from others in a similar state, and second to retain the capacity to think out effective professional responses of a sort that will also enlist the co-operation of these others; in the full knowledge that the consequences of misjudgement may be damaging, even lethal, to the others for whom he is responsible. Both need professional egos (to use Enid Balint's term) which are strong enough to withstand and not be overwhelmed by major tensions and which can simultaneously preserve full common sense and professional skills; all this without resort to pathological defences.

This is an ideal state which your Society seeks to promote and maintain by seminars following Michael Balint's pedagogic break-through. Yet, we know that it is achievable only intermittently and when the doctor is in good shape, and that failures are common. None of us dares be superior about this but it is important for furtherance of technique that we freely recognise failures of the professional ego when these occur, not to reprove but in order to study their nature, the circumstances under which they arise, the defences used against anxiety and the clinical consequences of these. By defences I mean attitudinal, social, geographic or tempo-ral changes and manoeuvres which, no matter how common or medically hallowed, can be seen to have been devised primarily out of the doctor's need to diminish his anxiety rather than primarily for the patient's welfare. But now for two contrasting examples of high and low defences in doctors dealing with a sense of helplessness.

The first doctor reported a year's events in a follow-up study. A middle-aged, married, childless woman, a steadily miserable complainer over the last 8 years, took to her bed after a fall and was still there complaining 2 weeks after, despite negative find-ings including X-ray. The solicitous husband had now called the doctor in yet again, and this doctor, usually mild-mannered and patient with her, now shocked himself by flagrantly bullying the patient. 'There is nothing wrong with you! You are perfectly all right! You are just complaining about nothing!' and with this vigorous reassurance he had stamped out.

Of course there was a long story behind this meeting of an unhappy patient and a doctor helpless and angry. For 8 years this woman had troubled her doctor with her miseries. He ascribed these to her mother who had lived with the couple ever since their marriage nearly 30 years ago. The patient never stopped telling the doctor about mother, how vicious and unpleasant, always getting at her, always saying she never had been any good, always saying her cooking was no good, etc., etc. The patient, unkempt, miserable and unsure of herself, had ups and downs. At her worst she could not face people, and the husband would bring her to the doctor by car and sit in it with her outside the surgery until her turn came. The doctor had felt for years that it was hopeless because the mother refused to budge. Then 2 years ago the situation had changed. Following a major row between mother and husband, the doctor had called in a geriatrician, the old woman was admitted to hospital and therefrom was discharged to a flat the husband had arranged for her.

The doctor, content that the mother's unpleasantness had caused the miseries, now expected his patient to be better, but she was little benefited. The doctor had attended and investigated her carefully after her fall and had found nothing. Nor had the hospital where he had sent her for X-rays. She had no reason to complain but went on doing so and her husband also expected the doctor to help her complaints. The doctor felt berated and yet helpless for there were no findings. Thus, unable to understand why she complained, he could not tolerate her complaining and told her she was complaining about nothing. The strain of being helpless in the face of external discontents overwhelmed his professional ego. In this attack he was denying to himself not only his ignorance and helplessness but also her need for any help at all.

Of course there is more to this case but because it is hardly relevant to my topic, I offer only a summary. Subsequent X-ray at a different hospital showed healing fractures of the pelvis. Her depression was openly recognised but not investigated. Several other matters have also not been investigated; her lengthy inability to assert against mother, her own right to have a home of her own, her childless invalidism in the marriage, her view of herself as a suffering victim, why the husband works regularly away from home and why he took over two decades to row effectively with his mother-in-law. But these investigations may never be made: the patient on a small daily dose of antidepressant, is now 'bright as a button', colourful and active, able to visit her mother and tolerate her nagging.

Returning to the doctor's loss of temper, it is known from other case discussions that he can be deeply moved by tragedy, but in order to keep his professional work from being affected he likes to be cheerful and unmoved and restrict his imagination in the face of trouble. Like all of us, this conscientious doctor shies away from lifting more than he can carry, and if he is in danger of feeling more than he can cope with he takes avoiding measures. In this he is like the rest of us. All of us have weak spots and against intolerably painful encounters it is inevitable that defences are erected, laughter, forgetfulness, aloofness, scotomata, denial and so forth. These allow the survival of the doctor but at cost to his effectiveness and the clinical results can of course be deplorable. This doctor's defences against involvement with the woman and the question of why she had to suffer so much were ordinary enough – evasive professional cheerfulness, concentration on somatic troubles or on the environment, plus reassurance. Her pains about the pelvis were the last straw, hence the denial of their validity and his firm reassurance about nothing to worry about.

The case makes clear yet again that all reassurance can be roughly translated as follows: 'Please stop being the way you are. I don't understand you and I don't know what to do and I can't stand being useless. I do not want to observe any more facts that disturb me. Therefore they do not exist. So please stop complaining. Now, look, I really mean it! So watch it! For God's sake keep quiet! Never heard of baby battering?* Shut up! Go to hell! My dear!'

My second case of hopeless trouble is told in extracts from the transcripts of the doctor's report to the seminar. The doctor is again a man:

> This started as a telephone call. Would I speak to Mr B. I said 'Hello Sid, how are things?' He said 'Oh blimey, doctor, fucking awful, Oh Christ, can you look in to see me?' I said 'OK Sid'. I made this the first visit. I arrived at a row of Victorian terraced houses, knocked and Sid, who is 83, came to the door. He said 'Hello, doctor, mate, come in, nice to see you' and I went in to see the patient, his sister. She is 89, is totally deaf – to me anyway – totally blind and she occu-

---

*There was an old woman who lived in a shoe
She had so many children she didn't known what to do
She gave them some soup without any bread
And whipped them all soundly
And sent them to bed

pies the front room. She is always in bed and was sitting now rocking herself from side to side and groaning 'Please, someone, help me'. I said to Sid 'How long has she been doing this?' and he said 'All bloody night, mate. Poor old cow'. I tried to say 'How are you dear?' and then Sid manages to get through to her, 'IT'S THE DOCTOR, DOLL!' and she said in a very distorted voice 'Who is it? Who is it? Where are you, doctor?' I said 'I'm in front of you, here' and put my hand on hers. With that she kissed my hand and held it to her face and cried quite profusely. Sid stood behind her and he was crying, tears running down his face, and he was saying 'Poor old fucking cow' over her head and I was saying 'Yes'.

I listened to her heart and her chest. Physical diagnoses have been many and varied: congestive failure, query myxoedema, blind, deaf. She has been in hospital a couple of times and come back with a series of diagnoses: and at the bottom of the form 'Social problem Y.7792'. It did not feel like that this morning.

Her deafness has been progressive. The blindness came on rapidly. Several years ago she was complaining of loss of vision and I sent her to the hospital as an emergency and had a battle. I would write saying 'Desperately urgent, increasing blindness' and would get letters back saying 'Thank you so much for referring this patient, there is nothing abnormal, we will see her in 1 year'! I would write again 'Getting more blind!'. I was put off by their negative findings and thought it might have been hysterical but that would not wash. Eventually they said 'Totally blind. Degenerative retinal changes'. I do not believe in the query myxoedema.

She stopped groaning and said: 'You've always been so kind to me, looked after me'. Which is not true – I have been of very little use to her. Sid and I went into the back room. I told him to tell her I would give her some tablets to take because although I speak more loudly than Sid, he does it differently and gets the message through in his gravelly voice. Anyway we had a little discussion, bemoaning our situation in four-letter words in which I joined. And he said 'What can I do. I'm the only one that can, nobody else can'. 'Would you like her to go into a home?' 'Cor, blimey, doc, no, she couldn't stand it.' (She has been in hospital on a couple of occasions with bronchopneumonia but apart from this Sid has always done the caring and I go along.) I think it is this business of standing being complained at, that he complains to me about the awful situation.

As I left the back room to go out, I looked in again. Mrs E had stopped this awful agitated rocking and now there was no sound. Maybe she was right, in some way I had sort of calmed her. Then Sid said 'Thank you mate' and slipped me a pound at the door. 'Here y'are doc.' He always gives me a pound note for coming, and always gives me a turkey at Christmas and Easter. Sid seemed to be satisfied that I had been just to hear about his difficulties. The nurses don't like to come in because they don't feel they do anything. Also it's the most incredible battle to get her admitted; they simply don't like her blindness and deafness and no one else can cope with her. It would be difficult to get her into an old persons' home. He's quite right, he's the only one who could cope. And he does.

Was she in pain, or just unhappy? She says 'It's the pain, the pain starts here and goes down my back'. It must be terrible, but I can't reproduce her behaviour, it's terribly distorted. By the time we had gone through this union of three, with all of us in tears, or nearly, it was much more peaceful. I prescribed 10 mg of Largactil three times a day but I don't know if they have been taken. I stopped her treatment when she came out of hospital on digitalis and diuretics, because the desirability of prolonging this life is questionable. She didn't go into heart failure when I stopped them, but it would be better if she died. I see her about once a fortnight, usually as a result of one of Sid's phone calls and I usually leave it to Sid to ring up. I said 'We will go on as before' and that is when he gave me the pound note. It's folded up and pushed at me, a present, not a fee. It's very worrying because I think she could live quite some time. The prospect of her living even many months frightens me, thinking about her isolation.

Contrasting with the first, this case is of a patient, her relative and the doctor on a footing of trust and affection. All here squarely face the misery and the pain and all accept each other's hopelessness and freely share the sadness about their helplessness. Moreover, in spite of severe suffering, the patient has no resentment about an unfair fate. Nor is she dissatisfied with her doctor. She complains to him but not at him and he is not pushed to cure, only to care. He is very sad but reproaches neither the patient for suffering so disturbingly nor himself for being so helpless and useless. Two matters support him steadily in this: first, the patient is of great age and nobody could prolong her life for ever; second, she and her brother do not reproach the doctor for failure to cure – rather they are grateful for his readiness to listen to and share their complaints and their burdens. Indeed the case raises again the important question – is having the right to complain as, or more, or less important than the actual complaint itself? Even in a fatal illness such as this both seek no cure but tell the doctor their troubles and they need him to complain to regularly, and reward him, not for curing the complaint but for accepting their complaining seriously. The doctor, with some embarrassment, enjoys their love for him as a professional of care and in turn he loves them professionally as patients. I ought to say here that love in professional work* is largely unstudied and decidedly much less than hatred, which seems to be more respectable and less shamefaced.

Here then is hopelessness, tragic, sad and painful for the helpless doctor and his distressed patient. But it is without any of the remorse, resentment or despair of the first case with its discontent, its suffering resented, with the tortured doctor and patient, both angry at the doctor's helplessness and with other strains in the doctor–patient relationship.

The second case (Sid and his sister), was manifestly painful but not unbearably strainful for the doctor. Perhaps this is why his defences against involvement with the patient and her brother were so few. True, the doctor's comic way of reporting can be best understood as his method of defence against displaying open sadness in the seminar: but he seems to have been little defended clinically. We may suspect too that his professional ego was nearly overwhelmed by helplessness and that his private ego nearly got involved in the tragedy. But he risked this and could be involved deeply. We can only speculate about the questions – what was it about these old people which made them so easy to encounter and to love?

Both cases required of the doctors' professional egos tolerance of their own medical helplessness. Why was this possible in the second case and so difficult in the first? The matter cannot be dismissed solely as a matter of the doctor' characters; for each is quite capable of the feelings and deeds demonstrated by the other in the different cases. There were differences between the patients,

*This needs careful distinction from personal, non-professional love for which there can be no place in the professional ego. Professional love is sophisticated, progenital and non-sexual, without passion or completion: rather it is quiet and seeks contentment rather than need-satisfaction.

however, but these have not yet been pinpointed. With Sid's sister the reasons for the doctor's helplessness were fairly clear; he was not in much ignorance nor mystery about the patient and the reasons for her unhappiness. In the other case the reasons for the patient's pains after her fall were far from clear. In spite of effort and hospital X-rays the doctor was still mystified, ignorant, in the dark. And still the patient complained.

Unlike Sid's doctor who *knew* why he was helpless, this first doctor was in a situation *beyond his understanding* and he was thus helpless *in an unacceptable way*. He knew he did not understand his patient's miseries – her failure to improve as he expected when mother left showed that – and despite some praiseworthy efforts he still did not know why she was in pain. It is this *kind* of helplessness which leads to anxiety such as to threaten the professional ego with private feelings and it is in defence against this anxiety the doctor retreats from encounter and thoughtfulness.

The retreat from encounter saved our first doctor from the anxiety of helplessness, but at the price of crippled professional common sense. Loss of temper out of ignorance has of course never been unusual in our profession but to deplore it is merely a pleasant moral luxury fit for the rear headquarters; and will not make it go away. We have to ask why is this form of helplessness so severely disturbing to the doctor as to threaten his common sense?

The anxiety which arises from the helplessness of *not understanding* is, from birth onwards, the major driving force behind ego development and the formation of ego skills. Indeed, man's very search for knowledge has always been driven by this anxiety, this terror of not understanding and of thus being helpless. The need to replace helplessness by mastery, and the helplessness of ignorance by the mastery which knowledge brings, ultimately animates all science. Man's search for knowledge and understanding of his environment and his self – yes, and of diagnosis – is thus fundamentally a defence against the anxieties which arise from uncertainty and ignorance. It is worth remarking here that some defensive manoeuvres – not all – can through later elaboration and adaptation come to have important secondary, almost independent, aims. But the embrace of knowledge is sought primarily to avoid fearful helplessness and to replace it with a sense of mastery. It is comforting to all; in medicine it is comforting to both doctor and patient that the doctor knows what the diagnosis is, what the prognosis is and what should be done and that he is a master of the situation, even when the diagnosis is grave. A doctor is turned to primarily in order to alleviate the anxiety of his patient's helplessness with his knowledge and skills; as we know, every clear diagnosis, even a serious one, brings marked relief to a situation which is panicky with uncertainty.

But who can the doctor turn to for relief when his anxiety, uncertainty, helplessness and ignorance run rife? There are particular problems in medicine about this. We are trained in objective methods; to examine, observe, elicit and classify symptoms and signs, to undertake special investigations, to sort out differential diagnoses and finally to arrive objectively at a scientific diagnosis for which there is usually a well-known prognosis and well-tested treatments. Over matters of bodily diagnosis general practitioners are therefore reliably competent and if, as on occasions, they are in great uncertainty, they have specialists to assist them and allay their anxiety. Yet this same scientific objective method has severe limitations as a method of arriving at all facts. Using the scientific objective method our two doctors could conclude that the two patients so far mentioned, once stripped of subjective emotional prejudices and involvement, were instances of well-known conditions: (a) reactive depression with a fair prognosis in a middle-aged female Caucasian; and (b) congestive heart failure with a poor prognosis in a senile female Caucasian. And that would be that. Objective science can certainly get at knowledge of things 'out there' *because* it eschews subjectivity but it is not wholly satisfying to practitioners simply because it *is* objective. General practice, like the whole of medicine, is not and can never be simply about an uninvolved, objective scientist meeting the objectified phenomena of disease. This is because a doctor is like his patient, inescapably also a human, being beset by feelings and wishes, by *subjectivity*; involved not only in the bodily fate of his patients and their lives as 'interesting cases or examples', but also in the other facts – that they are living, experiencing *people*, subjects of experience. He cannot ignore the latter without the major feat of mental blindness which produces scientific objectivity about living creatures; if he is not emotionally blind he will always himself subjectively experience something stemming from *their* subjective experience and react (by identification, reaction formation, placation, etc.).

When our patients are under strain we subjectively experience something of that (and react by identification, reaction formation, etc.), and no amount of ability to study, name and classify their strains in objective ways can set us at a distance from *our* experiencing something about their pains unless we use blind defences against experiencing something of their subjective strain. *Objective understanding itself involves, by definition, a refusal to reckon with subjective facts.* Thus, it contains a distancing defence against subjective encounter, such as our professional egos mobilise whenever our tension is too great to bear. I will return to that point soon, but meanwhile want only to emphasise the inevitability of strains in our subjective craft, strains which the pure scientist (who studies things and not creatures) need not experience nor notice. The strains of trying to understand the *distress of people* rather than merely objectively observing *pain in various conditions* can be immense; yet it is only by subjectivity with all its strains that we can experience our own lives and joys and pains, and the joys or pains and the livingness of others, and thus begin the task of understanding people and their troubles. Objectivity is safe and sure but very limited for the understanding of human lives, simply because it is concerned with people as instances 'out there', objects to be observed but not subjects to be experienced and felt about.

The trained, disciplined use of subjectivity as a source of scientific information is rare; in the service of medicine moreover it will inevitably often involve us in pain. We need not be surprised, therefore, and none of us can afford to be critical, if doctors seek ways of limiting their subjectivity and of alleviating the strains of uncomfortably close encounter; if they distance themselves from patients' distress in various ways, emotional, temporal, social and geographic; if they adopt and institutionalise as a profession various defences against the dangers of becoming helpless and stupid by having common sense swamped in big feelings about the distresses around them; and if they do their best to be fairly blind or hard of hearing or angry about distress.

Fifteen years ago when renal dialysis was at its beginnings and the country had only four machines, a keen young doctor was spending 8 hours each day with his patients who were on the machines. The patients were ill and afraid, and as he stayed with them monitoring their blood chemistry and physics they talked much and he got to know each of them closely. They had treatment every two or three days for a few weeks and he and his few patients became important to each other. They were children, students and young family folk, male and female. He knew their fears and loves and ambitions and they depended gratefully on him for their lives. He also got to know something of their visiting families. Yet in spite of his devoted effort the majority of his patients died, most of them while under his care, the others later at home. After the first six deaths, the doctor became less at ease with his patients and eventually morose, proper, remote and by the end of the year he was careful to have only a distant white-coated relationship with his patients and their relatives. At the end of his job he was apathetic about all hospital medicine and bitter about renology.* During the war I had found a similar withdrawn, apathetic state in certain tank commanders who had lost several tanks in action, escaping themselves from the turrets but leaving their comrades screaming as they burned and died inside.

It would be surprising if sure defences against such forms of helplessness were *not* enshrined in those medical procedures and attitudes of hospital life which keep patient and doctor at a distance ('Me doctor – you patient!). As students we inherited these safe defences in the *proper* routines of medicine. By and large these consist of the doctor making the patient fit in with his methods and timetable: an excellent defence against experiencing and studying the patient himself. We may therefore suspect

---

*It is interesting that when I came recently to check my facts with this doctor 15 years after the events, he at first said he had had many patients but few deaths. Then he slowly reviewed the figures. At first he denied that any were female; then he remembered the young women. Then he remembered the many deaths, how relatively few patients he had had, and how very few recovered. Last of all he remembered the children who had died.

history taking, questioning rather than letting the patient talk, interrupting him when he gets off the medical point; and when things get too free or he gets uncomfortably near to distress, switching to family history. We can wonder at why distress is so often classified under highfaluting names, why physical examinations are done at the particular moment they are done, and we can note how often the doctor may offer blind advice, admonition or wise saws or ideas borrowed from authority rather than thought out for the singular patient. And when we hear the doctor offering generalisations about human beings or reminiscences about cases and procedures based on nothing more than 'That's what I always do', we can be sure that we are meeting defensive security. For there is always a problem in doctoring – how much strain can one stand and yet keep one's capacity to think? The psychiatrist has a similar dilemma and indeed anyone involved closely with disturbed people faces it and has few choices. To be involved very closely with a *few* patients and share and follow major confusion, anxieties, despairs, fury and then work hard at sorting these out, to understand the patient's painful inner world and the unconscious relations he seeks of others? Or become a descriptive doctor, see many more patients, be cost-effective and kind but more remote or objective? Noting various sufferings only as important symptoms of the disease, and using similar distancing manoeuvres in treatments which do not involve the doctor as a person – physical treatments, community care, alternative environments, the social services? Perhaps move away from patients altogether; do research on biochemistry, or genetics, or the epidemiology of distress? Teach? Administer? All these activities, be it noted, *can* be important, useful – nay, essential. Defence against involvement with people is not to be condemned because it is not brave or because it is a sign of pain avoided. Rather it should be assessed – does it serve a real use, or limit potential usefulness?

All successful, rigid defence against the pains of human encounter means a loss of some capacity to experience something of oneself and the other. If sometimes the price paid for safety and the avoidance of any form of helplessness seems very high, it is worth remembering that defences are never there for nothing. The bigger the defence, the more sure one may be of the need for it. Again, how much strain can the general practitioner stand and yet retain his capacity to think? Every practitioner has a limit to what he can stand. He may be capable of making close working contact with a few patients in great distress (although usually in a schedule fixed as much by his ambitions as by his patients' wishes) but for the very survival of his professional ego he will then need defences against involvement with his other patients and he may be essentially a remote body-doctor with them. Another common way is to attempt sincere but less close and less regular contacts with all. Another is to wait, ready for, but not seeking, short, profitable contact with any patient, not now to a fixed schedule but only to seize advantage of a moment when the patient can reveal something of himself in a way the doctor can understand and respond to. This technique – the famous 'flash of mutuality' – clearly offers the least strain, for it only occurs if the doctor is ready and in good shape at the time.

We may regret that anxiety and defence against close encounter with distress is inevitable in doctors, but this does not mean that defence must be thoughtless. We can have some choices.

First, if we cease to be censorious about defences in ourselves and our colleagues as forms of cowardice, we can study and become conscious of the different *types* of defensive manoeuvre in common use. We can note the moments when they arise and thus be alerted to the half-conscious anxieties they defend against; and then we may consciously and thoughtfully estimate the nature of the doctor's anxieties and thus allow him second thoughts how best to deal with his anxieties about the patient's problems and to make fresh choices, deliberate and conscious now, about whether to encounter further or to defend. Thus we can hope to replace non-thinking, automatic, rigid procedures of careful encounter and defence by thoughtful, elastic and adaptive, deliberate techniques. If the doctor deliberately decides he must defend against intolerable strains then he may *choose* his defence and in full awareness decide which defence will be best both for himself and the clinical future of the patient.

Second, while continuing to value scientific objectivity in medicine, we may also avoid using it as a defence against the facts of subjective experience. The scientist deliberately defends himself against feelings about the object of his enquiry. Although too limiting in whole-person medicine, it has unshakeable value in the medicine of organs, as any surgeon or cancer specialist could prove. But if we dare value subjectivity also then we come to legitimise the study of the subjective feelings of doctors, the ways they at present are ignored in unconscious and undisciplined ways and how they *can* be used in deliberate and disciplined fashion to throw light on the patient and his problems. Thus we may open up a new field for study. Not even this Society has yet developed much science or deliberate skill about subjective responses in various illnesses and under various conditions (such as in February and July – 2 months when the doctor–patient relationships are quite different). Much of our medicine is blind and silent and frightened about subjective feelings; yet these are nothing new – they have always existed. They and defences against them have however been in *blind* use. What *could* be new is the deliberate study of their nature and ubiquity, in the hope of a more disciplined use.

Let me provoke you now by reclassifying a well-known syndrome in subjective terms: severe depression. There are various ways of classifying this, none wholly satisfactory, but now for a subjective classification based on living object-relations. 'There are two kinds of severe depression: those which arouse unbearable pity in others and those which arouse impatience and irritation.' And now for some questions such as might be asked in a students' examination. 'What are these differences due to? Which has the greater suicidal risk? The better prognosis? Which evokes tricyclic drugs and which ECT? And why? Is the comparative effect of ECT or tricyclics on each the same or different?' This provocation is merely to emphasise one point – that such subjective responses already blindly decide much of medicine. Yet they can be an important source of information and therefore a guide to action if they are respected and studied and not unconsciously and wildly acted upon.

One further simple example may illustrate the need for conscious subjectivity for doctors. A married woman doctor of about 30, a promising newcomer to a seminar, was consulted by a single woman of 28. She was 9 weeks pregnant and wanted an abortion. After 2 years of a steady and sexual love relationship, she had recently broken with her fiancé, having the bad luck of conceiving on the very last weekend of their engagement. She had thought hard about having the baby but had finally decided this would be foolish and unfair. Her own mother had been unmarried and, while loving and kind, had had a hard time bringing the patient up. The doctor, who has a baby of her own and blossoms in motherhood, liked the patient at once and the two of them got on well. The doctor, who has no objections in principle to abortion, followed the recommended abortion counselling procedure. Carefully and gently this intelligent doctor spoke about the risks of abortion – infection and perhaps lifelong sterility; yet made no reference at all to the greater dangers of a full-term pregnancy and delivery. She also asked about the fiancé's feelings now, but learned that there was no future in that relationship. He could not care less and would certainly not marry her. Then the doctor found herself asking an absurd hypothetical question: 'If you knew that this pregnancy was to be the last one in your life, would you want this abortion?' The patient was puzzled and talked round the question, but the doctor insisted – quite steadily – on it being answered. Yes, said the patient, she would still want an abortion. Now the consultation was faltering, so, feeling she needed time to think, the doctor told the patient to go behind the screen and get ready to be examined. Both parties had heard from the nurse before the consultation began that the pregnancy test was positive, but the doctor now examined and said 'Yes, she was 2 months pregnant'. 'How do you know?' The doctor was disconcerted but did not value nor think about that as an important subjective fact and recovering her poise simply explained the softening of the os. Back at the desk, the doctor suggested that the patient should think further about her decision, take more time, a week say, and then come back. Now the patient argued back; she had given the whole matter full, serious thought and had decided that she wanted the green form (certifying that termination should be carried out) today. There it ended.

The doctor now reported to the seminar that she had somehow made the consultation sound more strained than it had been at the time. It was really friendly and had ended without any discord (we may notice the doctor's need for harmony). Only during the seminar discussion did she ruefully tell that she had in fact signed the green form that day and the patient had left with it.

A medicine which valued subjectivity as a source of information would surely have allowed this keen doctor to be more observant about subjective facts, and surer about their importance and more careful to record them. Perhaps then she might have begun: 'Once we got on about mothers and babies my judgement ran out and I got dead keen for her to go ahead because I liked her. We gossiped like sisters but my weakness is that I cannot understand a woman like her not wanting babies. So I tried to frighten her into keeping it with tales of sterility. But that was no go. Then I wanted her to get married to save the baby but that too was no go. Then I tried to frighten her with ideas of future childlessness, but that was no go also. She just fought back so I decided to assert my doctorhood; I knew she was pregnant, but I did a vaginal examination just to let her know who's who. But now she treated *me* as a sister and we fought again. I wanted her to change her mind and told her to take time off and then to think the same as me, but she wouldn't. I hate open rows so I went on pretending that all was harmony and appeased her and signed the form. Peace at any price. So she got what she wanted, but I was fed up with her and sorry about the baby.'

If subjectivity was also *disciplined* the doctor might even have reported: 'I love babies, but I soon realised she was different. She charmed me and disarmed me and was very determined and I noticed that I found myself doing my best to like her but not managing it, and I tried to scare her. She told me a solid, hard-luck story of being both fatherless and now a deserted fiancée and no sleeping around. I'm not sure about this story. I noticed she was blameless and made me hate her fiancé (if he exists) and want to rescue her. But she only wanted rescue from pregnancy. Perhaps her story is all too good to be true. I am not sure how far she is suffering, but sure that she is a fighting type and although she provoked me into fighting back, I knew she would just get an abortion somewhere else if I didn't sign. So I did. At first I thought 'What a waste,' but then began to wonder what it was about? She's clever and able to get what she wants, and she's ruthless with her hard-luck manoeuvre. But what of her as a mother? She certainly made me so afraid of offending her that I appeased her.'

To conclude, your Society has honoured me by its invitation to give this lecture in the memory of Michael Balint. He was my analyst, teacher, colleague and friend and I hope I may follow his example and add to your burdens and interests. My suggestions are: that in your clinical seminars you become expert at recognising the defensive use to which any feature of an ordinary medical examination may be put, why it is used, when it is used and what its effects are on the patient; that you become expert at respecting and clarifying the anxiety of the immediate moment which evokes the defences of the moment and what part the patient has played in arousing these; that while respecting the need for defences, you become expert critics of any defensive manoeuvre that is thoughtless, rigid and automatic. I know you aim at these matters already. But, asking from the rear headquarters, do you know you do? Deliberately and consciously?

Finally, to escape from automatic and blind defensive procedures and behaviours, perhaps your seminars could make room for deliberate experiments in the fashioning and use of elastic, bespoke medical defences tailored for each case and each doctor. Your only danger could be the creation of new orthodoxies, new rigidities and new general rules. Yet I think you know that for each patient encounter there can be only one safe general rule, which is: do not have a general rule.

Index